T0251267

Outreach
and Care Approaches
to HIV/AIDS
Along the US-Mexico Border

Outreach and Care Approaches to HIV/AIDS Along the US-Mexico Border has been co-published simultaneously as *Journal of HIV/ AIDS & Social Services*, Volume 5, Number 2 2006.

Outreach and Care Approaches to HIV/AIDS Along the US-Mexico Border

Herman Curiel, MSW, PhD
Helen Land, MSW, PhD
Editors

Outreach and Care Approaches to HIV/AIDS Along the US-Mexico Border has been co-published simultaneously as *Journal of HIV/ AIDS & Social Services*, Volume 5, Number 2 2006.

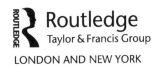

Routledge
Taylor & Francis Group

LONDON AND NEW YORK

Outreach and Care Approaches to HIV/AIDS Along the US-Mexico Border has been co-published simultaneously as *Journal of HIV/ AIDS & Social Services,*™ Volume 5, Number 2 2006.

First published 2006 by The Haworth Press, Inc.

2 Park Square, Milton Park, Abingdon, Oxfordshire OX14 4RN
605 Third Avenue, New York, NY 10017

Routledge is an imprint of the Taylor & Francis Group, an informa business

First issued in paperback 2020

Copyright © 2006 Taylor & Francis

All rights reserved. No part of this book may be reprinted or reproduced or utilised in any form or by any electronic, mechanical, or other means, now known or hereafter invented, including photocopying and recording, or in any information storage or retrieval system, without permission in writing from the publishers.

Notice:
Product or corporate names may be trademarks or registered trademarks, and are used only for identification and explanation without intent to infringe.

ISBN: 978-0-7890-3467-0 (pbk)
ISBN: 978-1-315-86436-5 (eISBN)

Library of Congress Cataloging-in-Publication Data

Outreach and care approaches to HIV/AIDS along the US-Mexico border / Herman Curiel, Helen Land, editors.
     p. ; cm.
     "Co-published simultaneously as Journal of HIV/AIDS & social services, Volume 5, Number 2, 2006."
     Includes bibliographical references and index.
     ISBN-13: 978-0-7890-3466-3 (hard cover : alk. paper)
     ISBN-10: 0-7890-3466-2 (hard cover : alk. paper)
     ISBN-13: 978-0-7890-3467-0 (soft cover : alk. paper)
     ISBN-10: 0-7890-3467-0 (soft cover : alk. paper)
     1. AIDS (Disease)–Southwestern States. 2. Community health services–Southwestern States. 3. AIDS (Disease)–Patients–Services for–Southwestern States. 4. Hispanic Americans –Health and hygiene–Southwestern States. I. Curiel, Herman. II. Land, Helen. [DNLM: 1. HIV Infections–Southwestern United States. 2. Acquired Immunodeficiency Syndrome–Southwestern United States. 3. Community Health Services–Southwestern United States. 4. Hispanic Americans–Southwestern United States. W1 JO671DG v.5 no.2 2006 /
WC 503 O94 2006]
RA643.83.O98 2006
362.196'979200973–dc22

2006018717

Indexing, Abstracting & Website/Internet Coverage

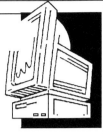

This section provides you with a list of major indexing & abstracting services and other tools for bibliographic access. That is to say, each service began covering this periodical during the year noted in the right column. Most Websites which are listed below have indicated that they will either post, disseminate, compile, archive, cite or alert their own Website users with research-based content from this work. (This list is as current as the copyright date of this publication.)

Abstracting, Website/Indexing Coverage . . . . Year When Coverage Began

- *(IBR) International Bibliography of Book Reviews on the Humanities and Social Sciences (Thomson) <http://www.saur.de>* 2006

- *(IBZ) International Bibliography of Periodical Literature on the Humanities and Social Sciences (Thomson) <http://www.saur.de>* 2002

- *Abstracts in Anthropology <http://www.baywood.com/Journals/ PreviewJournals.asp?Id=0001-3455>* 2006

- *Abstracts on Hygiene and Communicable Diseases (CAB ABSTRACTS, CABI) <http://www.cabi.org>* 2006

- *(CAB ABSTRACTS, CABI) Available in print, diskettes updated weekly, and on INTERNET. Providing full bibliographic listings, author affiliation, augmented keyword searching <http://www.cabi.org/>* 2002

- *Biological Sciences Database (Cambridge Scientific Abstracts) <http://www.csa.com>* 2006

- *Cambridge Scientific Abstracts is a leading publisher of scientific information in print journals, online databases, CD-ROM and via the Internet <http://www.csa.com>* 2003

- *CINAHL (Cumulative Index to Nursing & Allied Health Literature) (EBSCO) <http://www.cinahl.com>* 2003

(continued)

(continued)

Special Bibliographic Notes related to special journal issues
(separates) and indexing/abstracting:

- indexing/abstracting services in this list will also cover material in any "separate" that is co-published simultaneously with Haworth's special thematic journal issue or DocuSerial. Indexing/abstracting usually covers material at the article/chapter level.
- monographic co-editions are intended for either non-subscribers or libraries which intend to purchase a second copy for their circulating collections.
- monographic co-editions are reported to all jobbers/wholesalers/approval plans. The source journal is listed as the "series" to assist the prevention of duplicate purchasing in the same manner utilized for books-in-series.
- to facilitate user/access services all indexing/abstracting services are encouraged to utilize the co-indexing entry note indicated at the bottom of the first page of each article/chapter/contribution.
- this is intended to assist a library user of any reference tool (whether print, electronic, online, or CD-ROM) to locate the monographic version if the library has purchased this version but not a subscription to the source journal.
- individual articles/chapters in any Haworth publication are also available through the Haworth Document Delivery Service (HDDS).

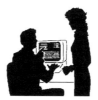

Outreach and Care Approaches to HIV/AIDS Along the US-Mexico Border

CONTENTS

ABOUT THE EDITORS

Herman Curiel, MSW, PhD, was Co-Principal Investigator (2000-2005), US/Mexico Border Health Evaluation Center at the University of Oklahoma, a Health Resources & Services Administration (HRSA) Special Project of National Significance (SPNS). He is Associate Professor at the University of Oklahoma School of Social Work and Adjunct Associate Professor at the OU School of Medicine, Department of Geriatrics. His research and publications focus primarily on minority issues with emphasis on Hispanic/Latino population concerns related to education, health, and HIV/AIDS. In 2003 he was the recipient of the "Care Award" for his ten-year Board leadership contributions to Care Point, a Consortium of AIDS Resources and Education located in Oklahoma City. He previously served on the editorial board of the National Association of Social Work journal, *Social Work*, and as consulting editor for the Council on Social Work Education, *Journal of Social Work Education* and the *Journal of HIV/AIDS & Social Services*.

Helen Land, MSW, PhD, is Associate Professor of Social Work at the University of Southern California. Over the past twenty years she has worked in the area of HIV, first in the early stages of the disease and continuing to be involved with clinical work, teaching, and research as the face of AIDS spread to people of color. Dr. Land has published widely on HIV/AIDS, with particular attention to the impact of the stress and coping process on physical and mental well-being in Latinas. She serves as a consulting editor of the *Journal of HIV/AIDS & Social Services* and the *Journal of Health and Social Work*.

∞ ALL HAWORTH BOOKS AND JOURNALS
ARE PRINTED ON CERTIFIED
ACID-FREE PAPER

Introduction

This volume brings together a number of articles that focus attention on the challenges of providing culturally-sensitive services to severely underserved people with HIV/AIDS in border communities, which include areas from Texas to California. Challenges abound due to language and cultural health-care beliefs and practices, lack of resources, stigma and fear of rejection from their communities and health-care providers on both sides of the border.

We are grateful to Herman Curiel and Helen Land who have conceptualized this collection and identified a variety of articles relating to persons affected by HIV/AIDS along the border. We are very pleased that the Health Resources Service Administration (HRSA) Special Projects of National Significance (SPNS) related to HIV programs in border areas are so well-represented. We thank Lois Eldred, Laura Cheever and Deborah Parham-Hopson for their support for these programs and the invited first article they provide in this work. Our hope is that HIV/AIDS agencies and service providers working with border populations may benefit from the literature and that the lessons learned from these communities have applicability in many other contexts as well.

We join Dr. Curiel and Dr. Land in wanting to acknowledge and thank the many reviewers that gave of their time and expertise to help produce this scholarly and important contribution to the literature on HIV/AIDS. We are indebted to: Dr. Barbara Aranda-Naranjo, Professor, Georgetown University; Dr. Morris Foster, Professor, University of Oklahoma; Dr. Gary Sinclair, MD, Assistant Professor, University of Texas, Southwestern Medical Center; Dr. Kurt Organista, Associate Professor, University of California School of Social Welfare

[Haworth co-indexing entry note]: "Introduction." Linsk, Nathan L., and Dorie J. Gilbert. Co-published simultaneously in *Journal of HIV/AIDS & Social Services* (The Haworth Press, Inc.) Vol. 5, No. 2, 2006, pp. 1-2; and: *Outreach and Care Approaches to HIV/AIDS Along the US-Mexico Border* (ed: Herman Curiel, and Helen Land) The Haworth Press, Inc., 2006, pp. 1-2. Single or multiple copies of this article are available for a fee from The Haworth Document Delivery Service [1-800-HAWORTH, 9:00 a.m. - 5:00 p.m. (EST). E-mail address: docdelivery@haworthpress.com].

Available online at http://jhaso.haworthpress.com
© 2006 by The Haworth Press, Inc. All rights reserved.
doi:10.1300/J187v05n02_01

at Berkeley; Dr. Shirley S. Semple, Professor, University of California at San Diego; Dr. Michael Tarter, Professor, University of California at Berkeley, School of Public Health; Dr. Michael Reyes, Pacific AIDS Education and Training Center and International Center on HIV, University of California at San Francisco, and Dr. Bernadette Lalonde, Northwest AIDS Education and Training Center, University of Washington. Michael Bass, MA, ACSW, Assistant Editor, provided expert editorial assistance and advice that helped this project come to fruition.

Nathan L. Linsk, PhD
Jane Addams College of Social Work
University of Illinois at Chicago

Dorie J. Gilbert, PhD
School of Social Work
University of Texas at Austin

Editors' Introduction

This volume is devoted to an informed discussion of HIV/AIDS on the US/Mexico Border and the unique dynamics of HIV/AIDS for border populations.

The HIV/AIDS epidemic in this region is made more complex by numerous factors including stigma, and political and psychosocial factors that influence Latino cultural perspectives on human sexuality. The rural nature of many parts of the border presents challenges for patients in overcoming distance barriers and managing privacy concerns. Further, it presents major challenges for administrators of health-care programs in recruitment of English-Spanish bilingual personnel who have expertise in HIV/AIDS and who are culturally sensitive.

To date, little attention has been drawn to the challenges of providing health-care services to people with HIV/AIDS in border communities. Importantly, little is known of persons living with HIV/AIDS in border communities. Latinos comprise 13% of the US population yet account for 19% of new cases of AIDS. Moreover, Latinos have the second-highest rate of AIDS cases among all racial and ethnic groups within the United States. The border area covers 2,000 miles from Texas to California and 60 miles North and South of the international border. Challenges abound in this area related to language differences, poverty, and cultural health-care beliefs that influence use of health care. Many people in need of HIV/AIDS treatment have no health-care insurance and receive attention late in the disease, or die prematurely. Others are hesitant to seek treatment because of stigma and fears of rejection by families, friends, employers, and health-care providers.

[Haworth co-indexing entry note]: "Editors' Introduction." Curiel, Herman, and Helen Land. Co-published simultaneously in *Journal of HIV/AIDS & Social Services* (The Haworth Press, Inc.) Vol. 5, No. 2, 2006, pp. 3-5; and: *Outreach and Care Approaches to HIV/AIDS Along the US-Mexico Border* (ed: Herman Curiel, and Helen Land) The Haworth Press, Inc., 2006, pp. 3-5. Single or multiple copies of this article are available for a fee from The Haworth Document Delivery Service [1-800-HAWORTH, 9:00 a.m. - 5:00 p.m. (EST). E-mail address: docdelivery@haworthpress.com].

Available online at http://jhaso.haworthpress.com
© 2006 by The Haworth Press, Inc. All rights reserved.
doi:10.1300/J187v05n02_02

Health disparities exist between men who have sex with men (MSMs), women, and children living with HIV/AIDS along the border.

This volume highlights HIV/AIDS articles that attempt to answer some of the concerns we raise. Five of the eight articles in this issue tell the story of projects that resulted from initiatives sponsored by the Health Resources & Services Administration, Special Projects of National Significance (SPNS) division of Office of AIDS. Lois Eldred, SPNS, Branch Chief, provides an overview of the five-year (2000-2005) US/Mexico Border SPNS initiative and how the efforts of the agencies, institutions, and individuals involved have resulted in lasting changes that better support the health care of this underserved population.

Two of the SPNS articles describe the populations and identify the issues that affect health care on the border. The first article, by Marguerite Keesee et al., uses statistical comparisons of Hispanic and Non-Hispanics; and the second by María Luisa Zúñiga et al. utilize qualitative study methods to understand border residents' health-care concerns within one region. In their article, Kessee and colleagues give characteristics of 1,200 participants in the five-year US/Mexico SPNS project that included patients receiving HIV/AIDS care along the 2,000 mile border from Brownsville, Texas to San Ysidro, California. This study helps us better understand the population living on the border and their health care needs. Zúñiga et al. present the results of a focus group carried out in San Diego, California that sought to identify common barriers that inhibit US/Mexico border residents from accessing HIV/AIDS healthcare.

Two other SPNS articles focus on models of outreach and training of general practice physicians. Michelle Valverde and Jennifer Felderman-Taylor describe an outreach primary prevention model designed to target high-risk groups living in border communities. Valverde and Felderman-Taylor's model of HIV/AIDS outreach, utilizes the traditional natural helper *promotor* model, using seropositive peers to reach at-risk populations in need of HIV/AIDS education and HIV testing. Gary I. Sinclair and Yolanda Cantu highlight a training model for health-care physicians, who work in border communities. The model provides information on supervision and consultation by an HIV/AIDS physician specialist who trains general practice physicians to care for HIV/AIDS patients in rural areas. The objective of this model is to expand HIV care capacity in resource-poor communities along the United States-Texas-Mexico border, utilizing existing Community Health-Care Centers.

Three remaining articles add important knowledge about Border population issues. Kurt C. Organista et al. describe an HIV/AIDS primary prevention qualitative pilot study with migrant Mexican/Latino day laborers in Berkeley, California. Patterson et al. describe a randomized controlled trial comparing an enhanced behavioral intervention, to increase safer sexual practices among US-Mexico border female sex workers in Northern Mexico, with a more traditional intervention based on Centers for Disease Control policy. In the final paper, Ramos and Ferreira-Pinto describe a "Transcultural Case Management Model," that incorporates the use of peer seropositive case-aid workers referred to as *promotores* who perform prevention and support activities for HIV-positive Hispanic patients.

This group of papers points to the common issues and interest that Mexico and the United States share regarding health-care in general, and HIV/AIDS and its prevention and treatment in particular. As a nascent effort to understand these issues and describe some promising efforts to address them, this compendium of reports can serve as a baseline for understanding the kind of research and health-care practices taking place at this time. Future researchers invested in studying border issues may want to build on these works and findings described here. Direct social service providers and other health-care professionals working with HIV/AIDS populations affected by poverty, medical care needs, and barriers posed by limited English proficiency and cultural differences, will benefit from studies reported in this volume on HIV/AIDS along the US/Mexico Border.

Herman Curiel, MSW, PhD
Associate Professor of Social Work
University of Oklahoma School of Social Work

Helen Land, MSW, PhD
Associate Professor of Social Work
University of Southern California School of Social Work

INVITED ARTICLE

Accessing Care for U.S./Mexico Border Populations Living with HIV/AIDS: The Role of HRSA's HIV/AIDS Bureau and the Special Projects of National Significance

Lois Eldred, DrPH
Laura Cheever, MD
Deborah Parham-Hopson, PhD

Lois Eldred, DrPH, is Director of Special Projects of National Significance; Laura Cheever, MD, is Deputy Associate Administrator and Chief Medical Officer; and Deborah Parham-Hopson, PhD, is Associate Administrator; all at the United States Department of Health and Human Services, Health Resources Services Administration, HIV/AIDS Bureau, Rockville, MD.

Address correspondence to: Lois Eldred, DrPH, Department of Health and Human Services, Health Resources Services Administration, HIV/AIDS Bureau, 5600 Fishers Lane, Rockville, MD 20857 (E-mail: LEldred@hrsa.gov).

[Haworth co-indexing entry note]: "Accessing Care for U.S./Mexico Border Populations Living with HIV/AIDS: The Role of HRSA's HIV/AIDS Bureau and the Special Projects of National Significance." Eldred, Lois, Laura Cheever, and Deborah Parham-Hopson. Co-published simultaneously in *Journal of HIV/AIDS & Social Services* (The Haworth Press, Inc.) Vol. 5, No. 2, 2006, pp. 7-13; and: *Outreach and Care Approaches to HIV/AIDS Along the US-Mexico Border* (ed: Herman Curiel, and Helen Land) The Haworth Press, Inc., 2006, pp. 7-13. Single or multiple copies of this article are available for a fee from The Haworth Document Delivery Service [1-800-HAWORTH, 9:00 a.m. - 5:00 p.m. (EST). E-mail address: docdelivery@haworthpress.com].

Available online at http://jhaso.haworthpress.com
© 2006 by The Haworth Press, Inc. All rights reserved.
doi:10.1300/J187v05n02_03

SUMMARY. The Health Resources Services Administration (HRSA) provides health-care to underserved areas in the U.S. and addresses disparities in health-care among U.S. populations. HRSA's Ryan White CARE Act provides HIV care and supportive services for persons with HIV and AIDS in the U.S. and its territories. Five projects were funded as Special Projects of National Significance (SPNS) from 2001-2005, to improve care and access to HIV services along the U.S.-Mexican Border. These projects developed culturally appropriate and innovative outreach strategies, expanded counseling and testing in border communities, assured continuity of care through intensive case management services and increased clinical capacity through provider training. doi:10.1300/J187v05n02_03 *[Article copies available for a fee from The Haworth Document Delivery Service: 1-800-HAWORTH. E-mail address: <docdelivery@haworthpress.com> Website: <http://www.HaworthPress.com>* © *2006 by The Haworth Press, Inc. All rights reserved.]*

KEYWORDS. Cultural, HRSA, HIV outreach, HIV services, Ryan White Care Act, SPNS, U.S.-Mexican Border

The United States (U.S.)-Mexico border region stretches over 2,000 miles and reaches across four states: California, Arizona, New Mexico and Texas. As delineated in the La Paz Agreement between the U.S. and Mexico, the border region spans 62.5 miles north and south of the U.S.-Mexico international boundary encompassing 48 U.S. counties and 88 Mexican *municipios/municipalities* (U.S. Department of State, 1983). Taking advantage of the relatively low wages of the Mexican labor pool, factories have sprung up along both sides of the border which in turn have increased the migrant stream of Mexican laborers heading north. High fertility rates in Latino families contribute to the rapid population growth along the border, which compounds preexisting social and economic problems. Approximately 12 million people currently reside in counties and municipalities along the border (U.S. Bureau of Census, 2005; Instituto Nacional de Estadisticas Geográfica y Informatica, 2000). In addition, almost 200 million vehicles and 50 million pedestrians cross the U.S.-Mexico Border at 25 points of entry (Bureau of Transportation Statistics, 2004).

Urban communities in the border regions struggle with pollution, population density and transborder populations with high needs and limited resources. Rural border regions face a different set of challenges. An estimated 400,000 people reside in more than 1200 *colonias*, small rural unincorporated communities that lack electricity, potable water, sewage and drainage systems. These conditions contribute to high rates of infectious diseases such as tuberculosis, hepatitis A, shigella, salmonella and cholera (Power & Byrd, 1998). Moreover, there is limited medical infrastructure with seventy-three percent (73%) of U.S./Mexico border counties designated Medically Underserved Areas and sixty-three percent (63%) Health Professional Shortage Areas for primary medical care (Bureau of Primary health-care [BPHC], 2000).

Given this deficit in public and private health-care, it is extremely challenging to meet the special needs of the over 90,000 adults living with AIDS in the four U.S.-Mexico Border states (Centers for Disease Control and Prevention [CDC], 2003). One role of the Health Resources and Services Administration (HRSA) is to address disparities in health-care among populations in the U.S. Since 1996, HRSA's Border Health Program has focused on the problems of limited health-care infrastructure, poor access to care, and poor health status of persons living along the border through several activities. Examples of HRSA's health promotion activities include the Bureau of Primary Health Care (BPHC) collaboration with the Border Vision Fronteriza project to train 800 *promotoras/promotores* (lay health workers) to enroll 15,000 children in Medicaid and the Children's Health Insurance Program. The Bureau also collaborated with the Environmental Protection Agency to train professional health-care providers and *promotora/es* in pesticide exposure, safe water projects, and asthma surveillance. HRSA supported "Ten Against TB," a screening project conducted by over 200 health-care professionals and *promotora/es* in the U.S. and Mexico working along the border to identify and control the spread of tuberculosis (BPHC, 2000).

HRSA's HIV/AIDS Bureau (HAB) serves the Border Region by providing funding for HIV services, clinical training and technical assistance to state and city governments, community-based health centers, and AIDS Service Organizations that serve border communities. The Special Projects of National Significance (SPNS) Branch of the HIV/AIDS Bureau funds demonstration projects to develop and evaluate health-care models to improve access to and delivery of quality HIV medical services. Since its inception, the SPNS program has funded a variety of activities to address challenges of HIV care in diverse settings. Recognizing the increase in persons living with HIV on the U.S.-Mexico Border and the challenges to their care, the SPNS program funded the initiative: "Demonstration and Evaluation Models that Advance HIV Service Innovation along the U.S.-Mexico Border," implemented 2000-2005. The goal of the initiative was to evaluate models of outreach and expansion of HIV specialty care delivery in this unique region. The Border Health Initiative included four community health centers, one AIDS Service Organization and one Evaluation and Technical Assistance Center. The participating service projects, across the four Border States were:

1. Valley AIDS Council, Harlingen, Texas
2. El Rio Santa Cruz Neighborhood Health Center, Tucson, Arizona
3. Centro de Salud Familiar La Fe, El Paso, Texas
4. Camino de Vida Center for HIV Services: Las Cruces, New Mexico
5. San Ysidro Community Health Center, San Ysidro, California

The projects formed networks of organizations in their regions through collaboration with a number of other community health centers, AIDS Service Organizations, county health departments, universities and AIDS Education and Training Centers. Each project employed a local evaluator to assist in development and implementation of the process and outcome evaluation goals for the demonstration project. The evaluation center, *Centro de Evaluación*, based at the University of Oklahoma, coordinated cross-site evaluation, provided technical assistance, and supported development and dissemination of information of findings generated by the demonstration projects. Unique aspects of the SPNS Initiative included the use of innovative outreach strategies, expanded HIV counseling and testing, and growth of primary care services through clinical training to existing health centers.

INNOVATIVE OUTREACH STRATEGIES

The Border Health Initiative developed a wide range of approaches for conducting outreach utilizing indigenous workers who shared common life experiences with the target populations. Migrant farm workers, cross-border truck drivers, sex workers, and trans-border day laborers were all part of focused outreach campaigns. The outreach approaches included personal contacts by *promotores* or peer advocates who share common beliefs and language with the target population. Spanish language radio, TV, and print media were used to educate the general public. The social marketing campaigns utilized educational messages to normalize individuals living with HIV/AIDS and to promote HIV testing to protect one's health and loved ones.

One-on-one outreach contacts were made by trained *promotora/es* at migrant workplaces, border commuter crossings and at neighborhood house parties convened for Mexican origin housewives. Truck drivers traveling between Mexico and the U.S. were provided HIV/AIDS information and condoms at truck stops known for sex worker contacts.

EXPANDED HIV COUNSELING AND TESTING

Each of the five demonstration projects established a unique network of coordinated services linking high-risk individuals to HIV testing, counseling and primary medical care services. San Ysidro Community Health Center improved quality of care by providing outreach staff CDC training to become CDC-certified counselors. In order to reduce the stigma, HIV testing was provided at outpatient general medicine health-care clinics in addition to health departments. Centro de Salud Familiar La Fe, at El Paso, recruited, trained and provided a stipend for peer seropositive individuals to provide support to newly diagnosed patients. Peer counselors worked with case managers to help patients link with medical care and other social services. Most projects were successful in their outreach work by providing HIV testing in venues where high-risk persons congregate.

CLINICAL TRAINING:
THE ROLE OF THE AIDS EDUCATION
AND TRAINING CENTERS

The AIDS Education and Training Centers (AETCs) Program of the Ryan White CARE Act is a network of regional and national centers that train health-care providers in HIV/AIDS care. As the clinical training component of the CARE Act, the program seeks to improve health outcomes for people living with HIV/AIDS by training medical providers on clinical management of HIV disease in areas such as use of antiretroviral therapies and prevention of HIV transmission.

HRSA's AETCs partnered with the SPNS U.S.-Mexico Border Health Initiative at its inception to support and provide clinical care training with the Initiative's service sites' staff, utilizing the project sites for local training. This element was critical to the success of the projects as clinical training needs were greater than anticipated. Both the clinical staff and personnel with non-traditional health-care backgrounds had limited experience working with HIV/AIDS and the affected populations, and had to learn the traditional medical aspects of care as well as dealing with stigma and other barriers to care for the population. Staff concerns included fear of exposure to HIV and misinformation regarding ease of transmission in the health-care setting, and attitudes about populations at-risk were potential interpersonal care barriers for health-care providers that required continuing education. Rural health clinics with limited resources had high staff turnover, which meant training of new staff was a continuing need.

CONCLUSION

Health-Care Model Created

All five demonstration projects identified above were successful in creating a health-care model that incorporated cultural health-care beliefs and the use of *promotoras* or peer advocates to link individuals in need of HIV care with health-care providers. The use of outreach activities like providing HIV testing where individuals at-risk congregate, the use of social marketing techniques to reduce public fear and encourage individuals to be tested, and the training of the clinic site staff to increase capacity and change attitudes were successful approaches as evidenced in the increased number of patients receiving medical services through these programs. The projects developed an innovative, culturally-congruent case management model to support a medical care team approach to providing comprehensive care for HIV-infected individuals.

Border Services Continue

The majority of these services continue to assure HIV care for persons living with HIV/AIDS along the U.S.-Mexico border. The funding supporting these demonstration projects made it possible for the development of a network of HIV/AIDS medical service experts within the region and at the state level. These networks continue to be instrumental in promoting awareness and advocacy to support prevention and treatment programs for persons living with HIV/AIDS on the U.S.-Mexico border via national and international forums.

More Border Information

The reader who wishes to learn more about these successful innovative approaches is directed to request a free HRSA video, "Innovations Along the US/Mexico Border–Models That Advance HIV Care" available at http://www.hab.hrsa.gov/specialprojects.htm. More information about the U.S.-Mexico HIV/AIDS Border SPNS program is available through the *Centro de Evaluación*: US/Mexico Border Health Evaluation Center at The University of Oklahoma at www.ou.edu/border.

REFERENCES

Bureau of Primary Health Care (2000). U.S.-Mexico Border Health. Retrieved on March 3, 2006 at *http://bphc.hrsa.gov/bphc/borderheatlh/default.htm*.

Bureau of Transportation Statistics (2004). Border Crossing: US-Mexico border crossing data. Retrieved on Nov 14, 2004, from: *http://www.bts.gov/programs/international/border_crossing_entry_data/us_mexico/pdf/entire.pdf*.

The Centers for Disease Control and Prevention (2003). HIV/AIDS Surveillance Report: Cases of HIV infection and AIDS in the United States, 2003 (Vol. 15). Atlanta, GA: US Department of Health and Human Services.

Instituto Nacional de Estadisticas Geográfica y informatica. (2000). Poblacion total por municipios y tamnano de locaida, y su distribucion sigun grandes grupos de edad y sexo (pafte 1 y 2). Retrieved on February 15, 2006 from *http://www.ineqi.qob.mx/ineqi/default.asp*.

Power, J. G., & Byrd, T. (1998). Introduction. In J. G. Power & T. Byrd (Eds.), U.S-Mexico border health: Issues for regional and migrant populations (pp. x-xviii). Thousand Oaks, CA: Sage Publications.

United States Bureau of Census (2005). 2004 Population Estimates, Detailed Tables. Retrieved on April 29, 2005, from *http://factfinder.census.gov/ servlet/DTGeoSearchByListServlet?ds_name=PEP2004EST&lang=en&ts=* 132770293125.

United States Department of State (1983). Environmental Cooperation: Agreement Between the United States of America and Mexico signed at La Paz. Washington, DC: U.S. Department of State; Aug. 14, 1983.

doi:10.1300/J187v05n02_03

Socio-Demographic Characteristics of HIV/AIDS Individuals Living and Receiving Care Along the U.S.-Mexico Border Through Five SPNS Demonstration Projects

Marguerite S. Keesee, PhD
Kimberly A. Shinault, MPH
Hélène Carabin, DVM, PhD
Ahmad Saleem G. Ahmad, MA
Kermyt G. Anderson, PhD
Timothy R. Brittingham, MSW

Lynda M. Williams, MA
Nancy K. Sonleitner, PhD
Adan Cajina, MS
Robyn Schulhof, MA
Herman Curiel, PhD
Morris W. Foster, PhD

Marguerite S. Keesee, PhD, is Program Specialist at the University of Oklahoma, Center for Applied Social Research.

Kimberly A. Shinault, MPH, is Graduate Research Assistant at University of Oklahoma Health Sciences Center.

Hélène Carabin, DVM, PhD, is Associate Professor of Biostatistics and Epidemiology at the University of Oklahoma Health Sciences Center.

Ahmad Saleem G. Ahmad, MA, is Program Specialist; Kermyt G. Anderson, PhD, is Assistant Professor of Anthropology; Timothy R. Brittingham, MSW, is Program Specialist; Lynda M. Williams, MA, is Program Specialist; Nancy K. Sonleitner, PhD, is Program Specialist; Herman Curiel, PhD, is Associate Professor of Social Work; Morris W. Foster, PhD, is Professor of Anthropology and Co-Director of the Center for Applied Social Research; all are at the University of Oklahoma, Center for Applied Social Research.

Adan Cajina, MS, and Robyn Schulhof, MA, are project officers at HRSA-HIV/AIDS Bureau.

[Haworth co-indexing entry note]: "Socio-Demographic Characteristics of HIV/AIDS Individuals Living and Receiving Care Along the U.S.-Mexico Border Through Five SPNS Demonstration Projects." Keesee, Marguerite S. et al. Co-published simultaneously in *Journal of HIV/AIDS & Social Services* (The Haworth Press, Inc.) Vol. 5, No. 2, 2006, pp. 15-35; and: *Outreach and Care Approaches to HIV/AIDS Along the US-Mexico Border* (ed: Herman Curiel, and Helen Land) The Haworth Press, Inc., 2006, pp. 15-35. Single or multiple copies of this article are available for a fee from The Haworth Document Delivery Service [1-800-HAWORTH, 9:00 a.m. - 5:00 p.m. (EST). E-mail address: docdelivery@haworthpress.com].

Available online at http://jhaso.haworthpress.com
© 2006 by The Haworth Press, Inc. All rights reserved.
doi:10.1300/J187v05n02_04

15

SUMMARY. The purpose of this study is to provide a description of personal lifestyles and demographic characteristics of 1,200 HIV sero-positive individuals who volunteered to participate in a Health Resources and Services Administration (HRSA), Special Projects of National Significance (SPNS) Initiative conducted in five U.S. demonstration projects located along the U.S.-Mexico border between 2001 and 2004. The results show that HIV/AIDS patients receiving care along the U.S.-Mexico border are predominantly Hispanics (81%) and men who have sex with men (56%). In general, SPNS participants appear to be socio-demographically similar to the general HIV/AIDS population in the U.S. with a few noted exceptions such as age, labor force participation, and variations in mode of transmission by age and gender. doi:10.1300/J187v05n02_04 *[Article copies available for a fee from The Haworth Document Delivery Service: 1-800-HAWORTH. E-mail address: <docdelivery@haworthpress.com> Website: <http://www.HaworthPress.com> © 2006 by The Haworth Press, Inc. All rights reserved.]*

KEYWORDS. Border health, HIV/AIDS, demographic characteristics, Hispanic, HRSA SPNS

BACKGROUND

The United States (U.S.)-Mexico border region covers four U.S. states (California, Arizona, New Mexico, and Texas) and six Mexican states (Baja California, Sonora, Chihuahua, Coahuila, Nuevo Leon, and Tamaulipas) and is approximately 2000 miles long (Bruhn, 1997). The population on the U.S. side of the border has increased by more than 300,000 between 2000 and 2003 (U.S. Census Bureau, 2004). In addition, it is estimated that 193,697,482 passengers in personal vehicles and 48,663,773 pedestrians crossed the border at 25 ports of entry across the U.S.-Mexico border in 2003 (Bureau of Transportation Statistics, 2004). The U.S.-Mexico border states include 48 U.S. counties (Migration Policy Institute, 2002), of which 24 share geographical borders with Mexico. It is estimated that slightly more than 65% of the residents in these 24 counties are of Hispanic origin with an average of 27% of those living below the poverty threshold (U.S. Census Bureau, 2000a; 2000b).

These 24 border counties do not have a well-established surveillance infrastructure, which limits epidemiological comparisons. Nonetheless, it has been estimated that 91,102 adults were living with AIDS in the four U.S.-Mexico border states at the end of 2003, of which 5% were in Arizona, 61% in California, 1% in New Mexico, and 33% in Texas (Centers for Disease Control and Prevention [CDC], 2003). The CDC estimates that among Mexico-born Hispanics living in the U.S., 61% of AIDS diagnoses in 2003 were attributable to male-to-male sexual contact (MSM), 24% to heterosexual contact, 13% to Injection Drug Use (IDU) (which includes combined risk behaviors of IDU and MSM), and 2% through other modes of transmission (CDC, 2003). These figures differ from those of U.S.-born Hispanics who reported contracting HIV mostly through MSM (40%), IDU (31%), and heterosexual contact (27%; CDC, 2003).

In response to social, economic and health needs arising from the rapid growth of the Hispanic population along the U.S.-Mexico border, the U.S. Health Resources and Services Administration (HRSA), HIV/ AIDS Bureau (HAB), Special Projects of National Significance (SPNS), funded five demonstration sites under the U.S.-Mexico Border HIV/ AIDS Health Initiative. The purpose of the initiative was to increase access to comprehensive HIV/AIDS care and reduce structural, socioeconomic and cultural barriers that may limit early detection of HIV disease among permanent and migrant residents along the border (HRSA, 2000). This paper provides a general description of People Living with HIV/ AIDS (PLWH/A) who reside along the U.S.-Mexico border and who agreed to participate in the SPNS program in one of the five sites between 2001 and 2004.

METHOD

Study Population. The target population consists of PLWH/As who were receiving primary HIV/AIDS medical services between January 1, 2001 and November 30, 2004 from any one of five HRSA, HIV/ AIDS Bureau, SPNS Border Health demonstration sites. The five SPNS sites were located in Harlingen and El Paso, Texas; Las Cruces, New Mexico; San Diego, California and Tucson, Arizona. Each site was randomly and arbitrarily assigned letters A through E to protect confidentiality.

Measurement Tools. Two uniform closed-ended data collection modules designed to measure information on demographic and lifestyle characteristics were used across all five SPNS sites. The instruments used in this study are available from the authors on request or at *http://www.ou.edu/border/*.

These modules were completed between January 1, 2001 and November 30, 2004 when participants were invited to participate in the study. The modules were administered through face-to-face interviews conducted by bilingual SPNS staff with participants occasionally completing some of the components on their own. Sites were responsible for interview training following the methodology and standards established by the collaborative. The consenting process and interviews were conducted in Spanish or English depending on the language preference of the participant. The questionnaires were originally developed in English. Professional staff at the University of Texas-El Paso, Department of Languages and Linguistics first translated the study instruments into Spanish and then back translated into English. At the end of the study period a second back translation was conducted by a Spanish speaker who closely resembled the socio-demographic characteristics of the study participants to ensure consistency in meaning and congruence in responses between Spanish and English items. Variables with inconsistent translations between the Spanish and English versions were removed from the database. This second back translation resulted in the loss of several measures of Socio-Economic Status (SES) including education and total amount of household income.

The socio-demographic variables included information on age, gender, housing, work activity and sources of income. Behavioral practices were measured using indicator variables such as self-reported sexual orientation, most likely form of exposure to HIV, number of U.S-Mexico border crossings during the last 12 months, and use of traditional medications or herbs in Mexico during the last 12 months. HIV status was determined at entry into SPNS from self-reported stage of disease progression including HIV seropositive (HIV not AIDS or AIDS status unknown) and CDC-defined AIDS. A dichotomous "Yes or No" measurement format was used to determine use of traditional medications or herbs. The interpretation of the phrase "traditional medications or herbs" was left to the perceptions of individual participants. In order to reduce problems associated with participants receiving services at multiple SPNS sites, one data record was maintained for each participant, with modules completed at differing locations; and the record that reflected the earliest entry date into the SPNS project was retained and all duplicate records with later intake dates were removed from the database.

Statistical Analyses. We report descriptive statistics on most socio-demographic variables measured in these modules by ethnicity and site. Several variables were recoded for statistical analyses or regrouped to respect the confidentiality of participants (frequencies of less than five participants per cell are not reported). Differences between proportions and associated 95% Confidence Intervals (CI) were calculated assuming a normal distribution of the differences. Chi-square (χ^2) and pairwise tests of equality of column proportions (z-tests) with a Bonferroni adjustment made for multiple comparisons were examined to identify statistically significant differences between the five sites using the Custom Tables option in SPSS (version 12.0.0) statistical software (SPSS Inc, 2003).

Age was calculated as the difference in years between reported date of birth and date of the first face-to-face interview. Age was grouped into four categories: 19-29; 30-39; 40-49 and more than 50 years old. The number of years between self-reported HIV/AIDS diagnosis and intake into the SPNS program was calculated by subtracting the participant's reported age at diagnosis from his/her age at SPNS intake. The SPNS project allowed grantee sites to enroll both new and preexisting HIV/AIDS patients. However, a measure of prior HIV/AIDS health care was not included in the data collected. Assuming that the majority of participants diagnosed after or within one year of the implementation of the SPNS project had never received HIV/AIDS health care, a second analysis was conducted excluding all individuals who reported a diagnosis date on or before December 31, 1999. The second analysis was done to control for potential confounding effects or explore potential effect modification of veteran HIV/AIDS patients on determining timeliness of entry into care.

Marital status was coded as single, married/living with someone and separated/divorced/widowed/other. Hispanic group affiliation was coded as Hispanic or non-Hispanic. Gender was coded as male, female and transgender. For the purpose of this analysis, individuals who reported being transgender (10 male-to-female) were recoded to male. Employment status was collapsed into three general categories including employed (full or part-time), unemployed but seeking, and not currently in the labor force. The category of "not in the labor force" reflects responses indicating that participants are not currently seeking employment and includes retired and disabled participants. Source of income was collapsed into five categories corresponding to no reported income source, public sources (Temporary Assistance for Needy Families, General Assistance, Social Security, Supplemental Security Income, State disability, and Veteran Administration benefits), private sources (employer cash benefits, private insurance, wages/salary), family support, and mixed income (public, private, and family). Housing status was dichotomized into living in owned or rented house/apartment and other (someone else's house/apartment, transitional housing, on the streets, institutions, and others).

Sexual orientation was dichotomized into heterosexual and gay/lesbian/bisexual, due to low frequency responses in other categories. Responses to the sexual orientation questions of don't know, undecided or prefer not to answer were coded to missing for this analysis. Mode of HIV exposure was categorized as: MSM, IDU, heterosexual, and other forms (blood transfusions or tissue and perinatal). Individuals who identified both as IDU and other modes of exposure were included in the IDU category.

Ethical Consideration. The study was reviewed and approved by the institutional review boards of the five sites and of the University of Oklahoma. Informed consents were signed by each participant prior to enrollment into the study by local project personnel. Both English and Spanish versions of the informed consent were provided to study participants. If participants were unable to read, the consent form was read to them. Interviewers ensured that all participants understood the contents of the informed consent prior to signing.

RESULTS

A total of 1,200 HIV/AIDS patients receiving care in the five border sites agreed to participate in the study between 2001 and 2004. The participants were between 19 and 73 years of age at intake into services and predominantly male (1,003, 84%). Nine hundred and seventy (81%) self-identified as Hispanics followed by 194 (16%) as White non-Hispanic, 29 (2%) as African American non-Hispanic and less than one percent as American Indian/Alaska Native, Asian, Pacific Islander or Other. A total of 712 (60%) participants reported their sexual orientation as gay, lesbian or bisexual. Among participants of Hispanic origin, 812 (84%) were male, and 567 (59%) self-identified as gay, or bisexual as compared to PLWH/A estimates of 92% male and 66% MSM provided by the Mexican government's Centro Nacional para la Prevención y el Control del VIH/SIDA ([CENSIDA]; Minichiello, Magis, Uribe, Anaya, & Bertozzi, 2002; Sanchez et al., 2004).

The differences in socio-demographic variables between Hispanics and non-Hispanics are summarized in Tables 1a and 1b. Table 1a shows age was the only noteworthy demographic difference between the two

TABLE 1a. Comparison of Hispanic and Non-Hispanic Participants from All Five Sites in Socio-Demographic Characteristics

Characteristics	Ethnicity		
	Non-Hispanic n (%)	Hispanic Descent n (%)	Diff (CI)*
Gender			
Male	191 (83.0)	812 (83.7)	−0.7 (−.6.60-5.20)
Female	39 (17.0)	158 (16.3)	0.7 (−12.42-13.82)
Age (in years)			
19-29	25 (10.9)	191 (19.7)	−8.8 (−22.26-4.66)
30-39	92 (40.0)	413 (42.6)	−2.6 (−13.69-8.49)
40-49	82 (35.7)	253 (26.1)	9.6 (−2.1-21.30)
50 +	31 (13.5)	113 (11.7)	1.8 (−11.61-15.21)
Marital Status			
Single	120 (52.4)	542 (56.1)	−3.7 (−13.69-6.16)
Married/live with someone	69 (30.1)	282 (29.2)	0.9 (−11.15-12.95)
Separated/Divorced/ Widowed/Other	40 (17.5)	142 (14.7)	2.8 (−10.34-15.94)
Employment Status			
Employed at some level	65 (28.3)	369 (38.0)	−9.7 (−21.72-2.32)
Unemployed but seeking	40 (17.4)	203 (20.9)	−3.5 (−16.51-9.51)
Not in Labor Force (including retired and disabled)	125 (54.4)	398 (41.0)	13.4 (3.42-23.38)

*Indicates difference in proportion between Hispanic and Non-Hispanic participants with a 95% confidence interval.

TABLE 1b. Comparison of Hispanic and Non-Hispanic Participants from All Five Sites in Socio-Demographic Characteristics

Characteristics	Ethnicity		
	Non-Hispanic n (%)	Hispanic Descent n (%)	Diff (CI)*
Source(s) of Income			
Income source reported as none	50 (21.7)	258 (26.6)	−4.9 (−17.53-7.73)
Public source(s) only	91 (39.6)	201 (20.7)	18.9 (7.4-30.4)
Private source(s) only	61 (26.5)	382 (39.4)	−12.9 (−25.01-−0.79)
Family	16 (7.0)	92 (9.5)	−2.5 (−16.36-11.36)
Mix	12 (5.2)	37 (3.8)	1.4 (−12.59-15.39)
Miles Traveled to Program			
0 to 4 miles	68 (29.6)	190 (19.6)	10.0 (−2.23-22.23)
5 to 11 miles	67 (29.1)	296 (30.5)	−1.4 (−13.48-10.68)
12 to 29 miles	33 (14.4)	261 (26.9)	−12.5 (−25.63-0.63)
30 or more miles	62 (27.0)	223 (23.0)	4.0 (−8.35-16.35)
Housing			
Buying or renting own house/apartment	112 (48.9)	453 (46.9)	2.0 (−8.34-12.34)
Other	117 (51.1)	513 (53.1)	−2.0 (−12.03-8.03)

*Indicates difference in proportion between Hispanic and Non-Hispanic participants with a 95% confidence interval.

groups as a higher proportion of Hispanics were in the 19-29 year age group (Hispanic: 191, 20%, non-Hispanic: 25, 11%), even though this difference was not statistically significant. This tendency did, however, follow the general demographic trends for Hispanics in the U.S. A larger proportion of non-Hispanics reported not being in the labor force (Hispanic: 398, 41%, non-Hispanic: 125, 54%). Table 1b shows that receipt of private sources of income was higher for Hispanics than for non-Hispanics (Hispanic: 382, 39%, non-Hispanic: 61, 26%). There was also a tendency for Hispanics to travel a little further to get care than for non-Hispanics.

Tables 1c and 1d summarize the differences between Hispanics and non-Hispanics as related to lifestyle behaviors. The distribution of sexual orientation and mode of exposure was similar between Hispanics and non-Hispanics, both among males and females. Slightly less than

TABLE 1c. Comparison of Hispanic and Non-Hispanic Participants from All Five Sites in Socio-Behavioral Characteristics: Sexual Orientation, Border Crossings, and Receiving Traditional Medicine in Mexico Last Year

Characteristics	Ethnicity		
	Non-Hispanic n (%)	Hispanic Descent n (%)	Diff (CI)*
Sexual Orientation			
Both Males and Females			
Gay/Lesbian/Bisexual	145 (64.4)	567 (59.3)	5.1 (−3.68-13.88)
Heterosexual	80 (35.6)	389 (40.7)	−5.1 (−16.67-6.47)
Males Only			
Gay/Bisexual	141 (75.0)	562 (70.3)	4.7 (−3.38-12.78)
Heterosexual	47 (25.0)	237 (29.7)	−4.7 (−18.38-8.98)
Females Only			
Lesbian/Bisexual	4 (10.8)	5 (3.2)	7.6 (−26.51-41.71)
Heterosexual	33 (89.2)	152 (96.8)	−7.6 (−18.55-3.35)
Border Crossings in Last Year			
None	107 (46.7)	200 (20.7)	26 (15.0-37.0)
1 to 36 crossings	108 (47.2)	477 (49.4)	−2.2 (−12.63-8.23)
37 or more crossings	14 (6.1)	289 (29.9)	−23.8 (−37.4--10.2)
Received Traditional Medications or Herbs in Mexico within Last Year			
No	221 (96.5)	810 (83.9)	12.6 (9.1-16.10)
Yes	8 (3.5)	156 (16.2)	−12.7 (−26.69-1.29)

*Indicates difference in proportion between Hispanic and Non-Hispanic participants with a 95% confidence interval.

TABLE 1d. Comparison of Hispanic and Non-Hispanic Participants from All Five Sites in Socio-Behavioral Characteristics: Mode of Exposure

Characteristics	Ethnicity		
	Non-Hispanic	Hispanic Descent	
Mode of Exposure	n (%)	n (%)	Diff (CI)*
Both Males and Females			
MSM	115 (50.0)	559 (57.6)	−7.6 (−17.61-2.41)
Heterosexual	56 (24.4)	289 (29.8)	−5.4 (−17.82- 7.02)
IDU including MSM and MSW	39 (17.0)	70 (7.2)	9.8 (−3.45-23.05)
Other (blood trans., comp., tissue, rape, mom to child, etc.)	20 (8.7)	52 (5.4)	3.3 (−10.5-17.10)
Males Only			
MSM	115 (60.2)	559 (68.8)	−8.6 (−18.34-1.14)
Heterosexual	24 (12.6)	156 (19.2)	−6.6 (−21.24-8.04)
IDU including MSM and MSW	33 (17.3)	59 (7.3)	10.0 (−4.51-24.51)
Other (blood trans., comp., tissue, rape, mom to child, etc.)	19 (9.9)	38 (4.7)	5.2 (−9.82-20.22)
Females Only			
Heterosexual	32 (82.1)	133 (84.2)	−2.1 (−16.76-12.56)
IDU including MSM and MSW	6 (15.4)	11 (7.0)	8.4 (−24.18-40.98)
Other (blood trans., comp., tissue, rape, mom to child, etc.)	1 (2.6)	14 (8.9)	−6.3 (−40.87-28.27)

*Indicates difference in proportion between Hispanic and Non-Hispanic participants with a 95% confidence interval.

one-third (289, 30%) of Hispanic SPNS patients reported crossing the U.S.-Mexico border more than 37 times per year compared to 6% (14) of non-Hispanics. Only 16% (156) of Hispanics reported receiving some type of traditional medication or herbs in Mexico, a proportion that was significantly higher than that of non-Hispanics (8, 3%).

Table 1e shows proportionately fewer Hispanic participants reported having AIDS (265, 27%) than non-Hispanics (86, 37%). Hispanic participants also tended to enter SPNS care earlier than non-Hispanics. Forty-six non-Hispanic participants (20%) reported entering SPNS care within the same year of their diagnosis as compared to 401 of the Hispanic participants (41%). The same general patterns persist regarding AIDS status and timing of entry into SPNS care when excluding participants who were diagnosed on or prior to December 31, 1999 from the analysis (unreported data).

Tables 2a and 2b show some notable differences in socio-demographic factors when stratified by ethnicity and SPNS site. Site A had the highest proportion of Hispanics who were employed (48%), seeking

TABLE 1e. Comparison of Hispanic and Non-Hispanic Participants from all Five Sites in HIV/AIDS Status at Entry into SPNS

Characteristics	Ethnicity		
	Non-Hispanic n (%)	Hispanic Descent n (%)	Diff (CI)*
HIV Status			
HIV not AIDS or AIDS Status Unknown	144 (62.6)	705 (72.7)	−10.1 (−18.66-−1.54)
CDC-defined AIDS	86 (37.4)	265 (27.3)	10.1 (−1.45-21.65)
Years DX Prior to SPNS Intake			
Intake within same year of DX	46 (20.0)	401 (41.3)	−15.9 (−28.93-−2.87)
1 to 3 years	38 (16.5)	214 (22.1)	−9.9 (−22.67-2.87)
4 to 5 years	27 (11.7)	98 (10.1)	1.3 (−12.11-14.71)
6 or more years	119 (51.7)	257 (26.5)	24.3 (13.97-34.63)

*Indicates difference in proportion between Hispanic and Non-Hispanic participants with a 95% confidence interval.

employment (35%), and receiving public (25%) or private (49%) sources of income. Site D had the highest proportion of Hispanic participants who were male (88%), 50 years of age or older (20%), married or living with someone else (36%), and who owned or rented their own house or apartment (67%). Site E had the highest proportion of younger Hispanic participants (ages 19 through 29: 26%), currently out of the labor force (54%), as well as provided care to the largest population of females (21%). Site C reported the highest proportion of single Hispanic participants (61%). Site B had the highest proportion of Hispanics who reported family as their source of income (14%), possibly explaining the lower proportion of Hispanic participants who reported owning or renting their house or apartment (35%). This finding may also be explained in part by differing economic climates associated with the geographic location of study sites, especially in relation to cost of living and housing.

Tables 2c and 2d indicate Site E served the highest proportion of Hispanics who self-identified as heterosexual (54%), while Site C served a higher proportion of Hispanics who self-identified as gay, or bisexual (69%) and who reported contracting HIV through MSM contact (68%). Site E also reported serving a higher proportion of patients who used traditional medications or herbs in Mexico within the year prior to intake (23%). Sites B and C served larger proportions of Hispanic participants who reported crossing the border 37 or more times per year (37% and 37.3% respectively) than sites E (14%), D (18%), and A (32%).

TABLE 2a. Socio-Demographic Information for Hispanic and Non-Hispanic Participants by Site

Characteristics	Site A		Site B		Site C		Site D		Site E	
	Non-Hisp. %	Hisp. %	Non-Hisp. %	Hisp. %	Non-Hisp. %	Hisp. %	Non-Hisp. %	Hisp. %	Non-Hisp. %	Hisp. %
Gender	N = 63	N = 63	N = 57	N = 296	N = 34	N = 311	N = 44	N = 50	N = 32	N = 250
Male	88.9	79.4	75.4	84.1	79.4	87.5	88.6	88.0	81.3	78.8
Female	11.1	20.6	24.6	15.9	20.6	12.5	11.4	12.0	18.8	21.2
Age (in years)	N = 63	N = 63	N = 57	N = 296	N = 34	N = 311	N = 44	N = 50	N = 32	N = 250
19-29	7.9	14.3	10.5	21.3	11.8	14.8	6.8	14.0	21.9	26.4
30-39	33.3	49.2	40.4	46.3	47.1	40.5	38.6	42.0	46.9	39.2
40-49	39.7	23.8	36.8	24.0	29.4	30.9	43.2	24.0	21.9	23.6
50 +	19.05	12.7	12.3	8.5	11.8	13.8	11.4	20.0	9.4	10.8
Marital Status	N = 63	N = 63	N = 57	N = 295	N = 34	N = 311	N = 44	N = 50	N = 31	N = 247
Single	58.7	55.6	45.6	57.0	41.2	61.1	52.3	50.0	64.5	50.2
Married/live with someone	33.3	30.2	35.1	32.9	29.4	22.2	31.8	36.0	12.9	32.0
Separated/Divorced/ Widowed/Other	7.9	14.3	19.3	10.2	29.4	16.7	15.9	14.0	22.6	17.8
Employment Status	N = 63	N = 63	N = 57	N = 296	N = 34	N = 311	N = 44	N = 50	N = 32	N = 250
Employed at some level	30.2	47.6	29.8	39.9	29.4	42.8	34.1	38.0	12.5	27.6
Unemployed but seeking	17.5	34.9	14.0	21.6	29.4	22.5	11.4	24.0	18.8	18.4
Not in Labor Force (including retired and disabled)	52.4	34.9	56.1	38.5	41.2	34.7	54.6	38.0	68.8	54.0

Non-Hisp. refers to Non-Hispanics while Hisp. refers to Hispanic participants.

Hispanic participants receiving care through Site D were less likely to report crossing the U.S.-Mexico border in the past year (32%).

Table 2e shows that Site E had the lowest proportion of Hispanics with self-reported AIDS (16%) and the highest proportion of Hispanics entering SPNS care within one year of diagnosis (64%). This contrasts with Hispanics in Site D who had the highest proportion of self-reported AIDS cases (40%) and diagnoses six or more years prior to SPNS intake (40%). Yet, for both Sites D and E, almost half of the participants had to travel 30 miles or more for their care (Table 2b). After reanalyzing the data by excluding participants who were diagnosed prior to or on December 31, 1999, this same general pattern of differences between sites remained with the exception that Site B now had a similar proportion of

TABLE 2b. Socio-Demographic Information for Hispanic and Non-Hispanic Participants by Site

Characteristics	Site A		Site B		Site C		Site D		Site E	
	Non-Hisp. %	Hisp. %	Non-Hisp. %	Hisp. %	Non-Hisp. %	Hisp. %	Non-Hisp. %	Hisp. %	Non-Hisp. %	Hisp. %
Source(s) of Income	N = 63	N = 63	N = 57	N = 296	N = 34	N = 311	N = 44	N = 50	N = 32	N = 250
Income source reported as none	20.6	14.3	26.3	27.4	8.8	16.1	11.4	32.0	43.8	40.8
Public source(s) only	38.1	25.4	31.6	17.9	41.2	21.5	50.0	22.0	41.6	21.6
Private source(s) only	31.7	49.2	24.6	38.5	29.4	44.1	29.5	34.0	12.5	33.2
Family	6.3	7.9	10.5	14.5	14.7	11.3	2.3	4.0	0.0	2.8
Mix	3.2	3.2	7.0	1.7	5.9	7.1	6.8	8.0	3.1	1.6
Miles Traveled to Program	N = 63	N = 63	N = 57	N = 296	N = 34	N = 311	N = 44	N = 50	N = 32	N = 250
0 to 4 miles	28.6	14.3	33.3	32.1	20.6	18.0	38.6	16.0	21.9	8.8
5 to 11 miles	15.9	11.1	40.4	33.1	44.1	47.0	25.0	18.0	25.0	14.4
12 to 29 miles	7.9	19.1	19.3	28.0	25.5	29.9	4.6	2.0	18.8	28.8
30 or more miles	47.6	55.6	7.0	6.8	8.8	5.1	31.8	64.0	34.4	48.0
Housing	N = 63	N = 62	N = 57	N = 295	N = 34	N = 311	N = 44	N = 50	N = 31	N = 247
Buying or renting own house/ apartment	55.6	61.3	15.8	34.9	58.8	46.6	70.5	66.0	54.8	54.3
Other	44.4	38.7	4.2	65.1	41.2	53.4	29.5	34.0	45.2	45.7

Non-Hisp. refers to Non-Hispanics while Hisp. refers to Hispanic participants.

participants entering SPNS care within the same year of diagnosis as Site E (unreported data).

DISCUSSION

This study is the first report on a population of HIV/AIDS patients receiving care at five SPNS sites located along the U.S.-Mexico border. The demographic characteristics of our study population are ethnically and socioeconomically similar to the population living along the border except for sexual orientation which is comparable to estimates generated from Mexico's HIV/AIDS Surveillance system (Minichiello et al., 2002; Sanchez et al., 2004). The population under care was 81% Hispanic which is slightly higher than the estimated proportion of Hispanics (66%) residing in the 24 U.S. counties sharing a border with Mexico (U.S. Census Bureau, 2000a). Among residents in the 24 counties lo-

TABLE 2c. Socio-Behavioral Information for Hispanic and Non-Hispanic Participants by Site

Characteristics	Site A		Site B		Site C		Site D		Site E	
	Non-Hisp. %	Hisp. %	Non-Hisp. %	Hisp. %	Non-Hisp. %	Hisp. %	Non-Hisp. %	Hisp. %	Non-Hisp. %	Hisp. %
Sexual Orientation	N = 62	N = 62	N = 54	N = 292	N = 34	N = 305	N = 43	N = 47	N = 32	N = 250
Gay/Lesbian/Bisexual	80.7	58.1	50.0	61.0	50.0	68.9	65.1	57.5	71.9	46.4
Heterosexual	19.4	41.9	50.0	39.0	50.0	31.2	34.9	42.6	28.1	53.6
Mode of Exposure	N = 63	N = 63	N = 57	N = 296	N = 34	N = 311	N = 44	N = 50	N = 32	N = 250
MSM	58.7	55.6	42.1	56.8	35.3	68.2	59.1	60.0	50.0	45.6
Heterosexual	15.9	34.9	38.6	29.4	32.4	19.6	18.2	26.0	15.6	42.4
IDU including MSM and MSW	15.9	9.5	14.0	7.8	17.7	6.1	15.9	8.0	25.0	7.2
Other (blood trans., comp., tissue, rape, mom to child, etc.)	9.5	0.0	5.3	6.1	14.7	6.1	6.8	6.0	9.4	4.8

Non-Hisp. refers to Non-Hispanics while Hisp. refers to Hispanic participants.

TABLE 2d. Socio-Behavioral Information for Hispanic and Non-Hispanic Participants by Site

Characteristics	Site A		Site B		Site C		Site D		Site E	
	Non-Hisp. %	Hisp. %	Non-Hisp. %	Hisp. %	Non-Hisp. %	Hisp. %	Non-Hisp. %	Hisp. %	Non-Hisp. %	Hisp. %
Border Crossings in Last Year	N = 63	N = 63	N = 57	N = 295	N = 34	N = 311	N = 44	N = 50	N = 31	N = 247
None	42.9	11.1	50.9	15.9	44.1	18.7	47.7	32.0	48.4	29.2
1 to 36 crossings	52.4	57.1	40.4	47.1	47.1	44.1	52.3	50.0	41.9	56.7
37 or more crossings	4.8	31.8	8.8	37.0	8.8	37.3	0.0	18.0	9.7	14.2
Received Trad. Medications or Herbs in Mexico within Last Year	N = 63	N = 63	N = 57	N = 295	N = 34	N = 311	N = 44	N = 50	N = 31	N = 247
No	96.8	90.5	94.7	83.7	100.0	75.2	95.5	92.0	96.8	76.5
Yes	3.2	9.5	5.3	16.3	0.0	12.9	4.6	8.0	3.2	23.5

Non-Hisp. refers to Non-Hispanics while Hisp. refers to Hispanic participants.

cated along the border, the proportion of Hispanics living below the federal poverty threshold (27%) is greater than that of the U.S. population in general (12%; U.S. Census Bureau, 2000b). Similarly 41% of our Hispanic participants reported not actively participating in the labor force and 27% reported having no source of income. However, it should

TABLE 2e. Demographic Information for Hispanic and Non-Hispanic Participants by Site

Characteristics	Site A		Site B		Site C		Site D		Site E	
	Non-Hisp. %	Hisp. %	Non-Hisp. %	Hisp. %	Non-Hisp. %	Hisp. %	Non-Hisp. %	Hisp. %	Non-Hisp. %	Hisp. %
HIV Status	N = 63	N = 63	N = 57	N = 296	N = 34	N = 311	N = 44	N = 50	N = 32	N = 250
HIV not AIDS or AIDS Status Unknown	58.7	60.3	71.9	65.5	64.7	75.2	43.2	60.0	78.1	83.6
CDC-defined AIDS	41.3	39.7	28.1	34.5	35.3	24.8	56.8	40.0	21.9	16.4
Years DX prior to SPNS Intake	N = 63	N = 63	N = 57	N = 296	N = 34	N = 311	N = 44	N = 50	N = 32	N = 250
Intake within same year of DX	9.5	28.6	19.3	46.3	20.6	24.4	13.6	18.0	50.0	64.4
1 to 3 years	14.3	20.6	15.8	23.6	17.6	24.1	18.2	28.0	18.8	16.8
4 to 5 years	6.3	15.9	15.8	8.4	14.7	13.8	13.6	14.0	9.4	5.2
6 or more years	69.8	34.9	49.1	21.6	47.1	37.6	54.5	40.0	21.9	13.6

Non-Hisp. refers to Non-Hispanics while Hisp. refers to Hispanic participants.

be noted that information was not collected on income sources in or from Mexico.

The CDC reported in 2003 that two-thirds of adults living with AIDS in the states comprising the U.S.-Mexico border were residents of California (CDC, 2003). Our data indicate that 67% of our study participants with AIDS were receiving care from service providers in states other than California. However, our data is limited to service providers participating in the SPNS project and is not directly comparable to statewide data. Grantee site selection was not based on the distribution of known HIV/AIDS cases in the U.S. or a random selection process; therefore the information presented should not be considered representative of the border region as a whole.

Our population is similar to the Mexican-born PLWH/A population described in the HIV/AIDS Surveillance Report regarding transmission patterns for Hispanics (CDC, 2003). Findings from our study indicate that 58% (69% among males) of the Hispanic participants most likely contracted the infection through MSM contact, 30% heterosexual contact, 7% IDU, and 5% by another source, as compared to 61%, 24%, 13%, and 2% for Hispanics born in Mexico, and 40%, 27%, 31% and 1% for Hispanics born in the United States as reported by the CDC, respectively.

HRSA funded this initiative to develop innovative models of care to overcome structural, socioeconomic, and cultural barriers that limit early detection of HIV disease among residents along the U.S.-Mexico border. We are limited in the extrapolations we can make from these data, especially on the effects that socioeconomic and geographic barriers may have in limiting PLWH/As from seeking care along the border. Limitations in our ability to extrapolate from study findings are due in part to the absence of comparative data from non-participants. The results from this study reflect the characteristics of individuals who were able to overcome barriers and obstacles to accessing care and willing to participate in the study. This study is not reflective of those who, for whatever reason, are not in care.

Comparisons among sites suggest that study Site E was statistically and epidemiologically different from other sites in the length of time that elapsed between original HIV diagnosis and intake into the SPNS project and level of disease progression for Hispanics regardless of the distance traveled to receive care. These findings persisted even after excluding possible long-term, treatment-savvy HIV/AIDS patients from the analysis, and suggest that Site E, a targeted AIDS Service Organization (ASO), may have been more effective at reaching the targeted population early in the disease stage than comprehensive service sites based in Community Health Centers (CHC) or AIDS Prevention Resource Centers (APRC). It is also possible that these findings are the result of confounding factors such as demographic and geographic characteristics unique to Site E's service area that have a sizeable influence on these measures. However, we believe the likelihood that the HIV/AIDS population varies substantially between these five sites in regard to HIV epidemiology is small. A more scientifically rigorous design is needed to verify these findings and the major contributing factors to the differences.

At the start of this initiative, HRSA staff and grantees hypothesized that delayed entry into care for Hispanics residing along the U.S.-Mexico border was a result in part to difficulties associated with crossing the border and the extensive distances a patient must travel to care. Our results contradict this belief. In effect, there was an important variation between sites in the distance that participants had to travel to receive care even though they may have entered SPNS care within a similar time span following diagnosis. For example, Hispanic participants from Sites C and D were both more likely to enter SPNS care six or more years after diagnosis than Hispanic participants being served at the other project sites. Yet, most participants from Site C traveled between five and 11 miles whereas most participants from Site D traveled 30 or more miles to the care site. Hence, for a similar lag time between diagnosis and entry into SPNS care, the distance traveled was very different. In addition, these care facilities were enrolling patients into SPNS care much later than Site E where a large proportion of participants traveled more than 30 miles to receive care. These same general patterns of timing of entry into SPNS care and miles traveled to the treatment facility persisted even after excluding individuals who reported a diagnosis prior to or on December 31, 1999. Furthermore, border crossings do not appear to be a significant barrier to accessing care for participants enrolled in the SPNS program. For example, an equal proportion of Hispanic participants receiving care at Sites A and E were likely to cross the border between one and 36 times per year, while participants receiving care at Site A were diagnosed much later than at Site E. At Site D, Hispanic participants were less likely to cross the border than other sites although they were likely to come into SPNS care six or more years after diagnosis. These findings do not provide support for the assertions that the distance traveled to service sites and the number of border crossings have an important impact on when PLWH/As residing along the U.S.-Mexico border enter HIV/AIDS medical care. Studies of migration patterns between Mexico and the U.S. have found that a large proportion of Mexican migrants who travel to the U.S. utilize well-developed migrant networks that provide social, informational and material support (Aguilera & Massey, 2003; Fussell, 2004; Kanaiaupuni, 2000; Kandel & Massey, 2002; Phillips & Massey, 2000; Singer & Massey, 1998). These networks may act to reduce the likelihood that issues associated with crossing the U.S.-Mexico border and the distance traveled to obtain needed services operate as barriers to receiving care. Additionally, some participants may consciously choose to utilize service providers located outside of their communities of residence in order to ensure their anonymity.

Another belief contradicted by our results is that patients with better financial resources are likely to seek care more readily. Patients at Site E were more likely to report no source of income than any of the other sites and yet, a larger proportion was seeking care early after diagnosis. Also, the tendency of Hispanic participants to report being employed and having private income sources more frequently than non-Hispanics suggests that non-Hispanics under care in the border region may have greater access to public sources of income (Ruiz-Beltran & Kamau, 2001). Moreover, higher proportions of employment and private income sources may also be reflective of the younger age distribution of the Hispanic population.

A recent Morbidity and Mortality Weekly Report (MMWR) (CDC, 2004a) estimated that in 29 States between 1999 and 2002, 64% of reported heterosexual HIV transmissions occurred in females. The proportion of females among heterosexual PLWH/As in our study population was smaller (48%). The CDC's definition of heterosexual transmission is more specific than that of SPNS. Specifically, the CDC definition includes heterosexual contact with an HIV-infected person or one at high risk for HIV infection through IDU, while the SPdNS definition includes heterosexual contact with an HIV-infected person (which may or may not be at high risk through IDU). However, we feel that this comparison is reasonable, in that both studies aim to measure the same parameter.

Thirty-six percent of heterosexual study participants diagnosed within one year of intake were in the 30-39 year age group, which mirrors the national estimate of 35% in men and women (CDC, 2004a). The report also states that, in women with HIV infection, the proportion that contracts the disease by heterosexual contact is highest in those between 13 and 19 years of age and steadily declines in older age groups. Conversely, our data show the proportion of self-reported heterosexual exposure is constant and lower than reported in the MMWR until 40 years of age, and subsequently decreases by half (unreported data; CDC, 2004a). Notably, a lower proportion of young women who receive care from SPNS providers located along the U.S.-Mexico border report having contracted the infection heterosexually as compared to national estimates. When compared to recent estimates provided by the CDC, females in the SPNS sample appear to be underrepresented with 16% of the SPNS sample comprised of women compared to an estimated 22% of the adult and adolescent PLWH/A population in the U.S. (CDC, 2003). One possible explanation for the low level of female participation is that outreach models were less effective in reaching at-risk female populations, such as those who do not perceive or acknowledge risk because of being in a monogamous committed relationship and a personal lack of involvement in behaviors believed to be associated with increased risk, than at reaching at-risk males (Hirsch, Higgins, Bentley, & Nathanson, 2002; Keesee, Ahmad, Nelson, Barney, & Duran, 2004; Newcomb et al., 1998). It is also possible that migrating females from Mexico who are following domestic partners or spouses are less likely to engage in stage migration, thereby bypassing border communities and moving directly to a predetermined final destination (Fussell, 2004; Cerrutti & Massey, 2001). Further research is needed in this area.

Between 2000 and 2003, it was estimated that 61% of men contracted HIV by MSM transmission in 32 States (CDC, 2004b), which is lower than the 67% (95% CI 64.2-70.1) found in our study. This suggests that among male PLWH/As receiving care along the border, more men are infected through MSM transmission than the national average (see also Hall, Li, & McKenna, 2005). The greater proportion of MSM transmission may be the result of a convergence between Mexican MSM migrating to the U.S. in search of less restrictive social attitudes and more permissive norms regarding sexuality in the U.S. (Díaz, 1998; Marks, Cantero, & Simoni, 1998) and the use of border communities by potential migrants as staging areas or a home base to collect migration-related information and resources for future documented and undocumented trips to the U.S. (Fussell, 2004).

Our study had several limitations. The first major limitation is the lack of a comparison group which restricts our description of socio-demographic and behavioral aspects to participants in our study and variations between the five sites. In addition, we were unable to assess the possibility of selection bias since data on refusals to participate in the SPNS project were not collected. Another limitation is that we were unable to report education and income levels for the study population due to incongruence between the Spanish and English versions of the questionnaire and methods of instrument administration. Finally, we cannot guarantee that questions were asked exactly the same way by different interviewers across sites. For example, it is possible that observed differences between sites were due in part to the use of different criteria for coding the variable "use of traditional medication and herbs from Mexico." Quality control information was not collected nor were interviewers monitored at all sites, therefore it is not possible to adjust for variations associated with potential measurement error and selection bias. One potential source of measurement error was interviewer turnover throughout the study period.

Nonetheless, our study population of PLWH/As receiving care in one of five sites along the U.S.-Mexico border provides insights and ideas for generating hypotheses to test differences between this and the general U.S. PLWH/A populations. The exposure risk factors of our study population are quite similar to that found in the national Mexico-born Hispanic population (CDC, 2003). This suggests that culturally sensitive prevention and outreach activities should be offered to all Mexico-born Hispanic men and women at various ages in the U.S., and that these should take into consideration the differing transmission factors in that population as compared to the U.S. born population (Díaz, 1998; Foreman, 1999; Keesee et al., 2004; Ramirez-Valles, Zimmerman, Suarez, & De la Rosa, 1998; Russell, Alexander, & Corbo, 2000). Further, our findings indicate that significant diversity exists between the Hispanic populations receiving HIV/AIDS health services along the border in the four states, which may suggest a need for adapted approaches to social service and outreach. Future research needs to include an assessment of the impact of structural, environmental, economic and social factors of border communities and/or regions compared to non-border communities on the risk for HIV transmission and on an increasing access to health care on both sides of the border (Organista, Carrillo, & Ayala, 2004). This population diversity also requires that future evaluative studies include a significantly larger number of service sites and a standardized set of prevention and outreach protocols.

AUTHOR NOTE

Address correspondence to: Marguerite Keesee, PhD, University of Oklahoma, Center for Applied Social Research, Parkway South, 3200 Marshall Avenue, Suite 230, Norman, OK 73072-8032 (E-mail: mkeesee@ou.edu).

U.S.-Mexico Border HIV/AIDS Collaborative consists of the program staff, project evaluators and HRSA project staff involved in implementing and operating the U.S.-Mexico Border Health HIV/AIDS Special Programs of National Significance initiative at all five project sites and the University of Oklahoma.

The special initiative for the development of Demonstration and Evaluation Models that Advance HIV Service Innovation Along the U.S.- Mexico Border is funded by the U.S. Department of Health and Human Services (DHHS), Health Resources and Services Administration (HRSA), HIV/AIDS Bureau (HAB), Office of Science and Epidemiology, Special Projects of National Significance (SPNS), Grant #5 H97 HA 00180 03.

The U.S.-Mexico Border grantee sites which contributed to the data base used in this study include: *El Rio* Health Center/Arizona Border HIV/AIDS Care Project (ABHAC)(Tucson, AZ), *Camino de Vida* Center for HIV Services (Las Cruces, NM), *Centro de Salud Familiar La Fe* (El Paso, TX), *San Ysidro* Health Center (San Ysidro, CA), Valley AIDS Council (Harlingen, TX) and the *Centro de Evaluación*: U.S.-Mexico Border Health Evaluation Center (Norman, OK).

REFERENCES

Aguilera, M. B., & Massey, D. S. (2003). Social capital and the wages of Mexican migrants: New hypotheses and tests. *Social Forces, 82*(2), 671-701.

Bruhn, J. G. (1997). Introduction. In J. G. Bruhn & J. E. Brandon (Eds.), *Border health: Challenges for the United States and Mexico* (pp. 3-12). NY: Garland Publishing.

Bureau of Transpotation Statistics (2004). Border crossing: US-Mexico border crossing data. Retrieved on November 14, 2004, from *http://www.bts.gov/programs/international/border_crossing_entry_data/us_mexico/pdf/entire.pdf*

The Centers for Disease Control and Prevention (2003). *HIV/AIDS Surveillance Report: Cases of HIV infection and AIDS in the United States, 2003 (Vol. 15).* Atlanta, GA: US Department of Health and Human Services.

The Centers for Disease Control and Prevention (2004a, February 20). Heterosexual transmission of HIV-29 states, 1999-2002. *Morbidity and Mortality Weekly Report, 53*(6): 125-129.

The Centers for Disease Control and Prevention (2004b, December 3). Diagnoses of HIV/AIDS–32 states, 2000-2003. *Morbidity and Mortality Weekly Report, 53*(47): 1106-1110.

Cerrutti, M., & Massey, D. S. (2001). On the auspices of female migration from Mexico to the United States. *Demography, 38*(2), 187-200.

Díaz, R. M. (1998). *Latino gay men and HIV.* London: Routledge.

Foreman, M. (1999). Changing men's behavior. In M. Foreman (Ed.), *AIDS and men: Taking risks or taking responsibility?* (pp. 36-49). London, United Kingdom: Zed Books Ltd.

Fussell, E. (2004). Sources of Mexico's migration stream: Rural, urban, and border migrants to the United States. *Social Forces, 82*(3), 937-967.

Hall, H. I., Li, J., & McKenna, M. T. (2005). HIV in predominantly rural areas of the United States. *The Journal of Rural Health, 21*(3), 245-253.

Health Resources and Services Administration [HRSA] (2000). Special Programs of National Significance: Report on new 1999-2000 initiatives. Retrieved January 27, 2005, from *ftp://ftp.hrsa.gov/hab/SpnsRpt5.pdf.*

Hirsch, J. S., Higgins, J., Bentley, M. E., & Nathanson, C. A. (2002). The social constructions of sexuality: Marital infidelity and sexually transmitted disease–HIV risk in a Mexican migrant community. *American Journal of Public Health, 92*(8), 1227-1237.

Kanaiaupuni, S. M. (2000). Reframing the migration question: An analysis of men, women, and gender in Mexico. *Social Forces, 78*(4), 1311-1348.

Kandel, W., & Massey, D. S. (2002). The culture of Mexican migration: A theoretical and empirical analysis. *Social Forces, 80*(3), 981-1004.

Keesee, M. S., Ahmad, A. S. G., Nelson, W., Barney, D. D., & Duran, B. (2004). An application of Borrayo's Cultural Health Belief Model to HIV/AIDS seropositive Hispanics living along the US/Mexico border. *Journal of HIV/AIDS & Social Services, 3,* 9-34.

Marks, G., Cantero, P. J., & Simoni, J. M. (1998). Is acculturation associated with sexual risk behaviours? An investigation of HIV-positive Latino men and women. *AIDS Care, 10*(3), 283-2297.

Migration Policy Institute. (July 2002). Migration information source: The US-Mexico border. Retrieved June 01, 2005, from *http://www.migrationinformation.org/feature/display.cfm?ID=32.*

Minichiello, S. N., Magis, C., Uribe, P., Anaya, L., & Bertozzi, S. (2002). The Mexican HIV/AIDS surveillance system: 1986-2001. *AIDS, 16* (suppl 3), S13-S17.

Newcomb, M. D., Wyatt, G. E., Romero, G. J., Tucker, M. B., Wayment, H. A., Carmona, J. V. et al. (1998). Acculturation, sexual risk taking, and HIV health promotion among Latinas. *Journal of Counseling Psychology, 45*(4), 454-466.

Organista, K. C., Carrillo, H., & Ayala, G. (2004). HIV prevention with Mexican migrants: Review, critique and recommendations. *Journal of Acquired Immune Deficiency Syndromes, 37* (suppl 4), S227-239.

Phillips, J. A., & Massey, D. S. (2000). Engines of immigration: Stocks of human and social capital in Mexico. *Social Science Quarterly 81*(1), 33-48.

Ramirez-Valles, J., Zimmerman, M. A., Suarez, E., & De la Rosa, G. (1998). A patch for the quilt: HIV/AIDS, homosexual men, and community mobilization on the US/Mexico border. In J.G. Power & T. Byrd (Eds.), *US-Mexico border health: Issues for regional and migrant populations* (pp. 103-118). Thousand Oaks, CA: Sage.

Ruiz-Beltran, M., & Kamau, J. K. (2001). The socio-economic and cultural impediments to well-being along the US-Mexico border. *Journal of Community Health, 26*(2), 123-132.

Russell, L. D., Alexander, M. K., & Corbo, K. F. (2000). Developing culture-specific interventions for Latinas to reduce HIV high-risk behaviors. *Journal of the Association of Nurses in AIDS Care, 11*(3), 70-76.

Sanchez, M. A., Lemp, G. F., Magis-Rodriguez, C., Bravo-Garcia, E., Carter, S., & Ruiz, J. D. (2004). The epidemiology of HIV among Mexican migrants and recent immigrants in California and Mexico. *Journal of Acquired Immune Deficiency Syndromes, 37* (suppl 4), S204- 214.

Singer, A., & Massey, D. S. (1998). The social process of undocumented border crossing among Mexican migrants. *International Migration Review, 32*(3), 561-592.

SPSS Inc. (2003). *SPSS Base 12.0.0 for Windows user's guide. SPSS Inc.,* Chicago, IL.

U.S. Census Bureau. (2000a). Census 2000 Summary File 3 (SF 3)–Sample data. Retrieved on November 14, 2004, from *http://factfinder.census.gov/servlet/DatasetMainPageServlet?_program=DEC&_lang=en*

U.S. Census Bureau (2000b). State and county quick facts. Retrieved on June 1, 2005 from *http://quickfacts.census.gov/qfd/*

U.S. Census Bureau (2004*).* 2003 Population estimates. Retrieved on November 14, 2004, from *http://factfinder.census.gov/servlet/DatasetMainPageServlet?_program = PEP&_lang=en&ts=131556701203*

doi:10.1300/J187v05n02_04

Exploring Care Access Issues
for Mexican-Origin Latinos
Living with HIV
in the San Diego/Tijuana Border Region

María Luisa Zúñiga, PhD
Kurt C. Organista, PhD
Rosana Scolari, BA

Alisa M. Olshefsky, BA
Robyn Schulhof, MA
Madeline Colón, MS

María Luisa Zúñiga, PhD, is Assistant Professor and Director of Program Evaluation at the University of California, San Diego (UCSD), Division of Community Pediatrics, San Diego, CA.

Kurt C. Organista, PhD, is Associate Professor at the School of Social Welfare, University of California, Berkeley, CA.

Rosana Scolari, BA, is Director of HIV/AIDS Services, San Ysidro Health Center, San Ysidro, CA.

Alisa M. Olshefsky, BA, is Evaluation Studies Manager at UCSD Division of Community Pediatrics, San Diego, CA.

Robyn Schulhof, MA, is SPNS Public Health Analyst, Health Resources and Services Administration, HIV/AIDS Bureau, United States Department of Health and Human Services, Rockville, MA.

Madeline Colón, MS, was an intern at Health Resources and Services Administration, Ponce, Puerto Rico.

Address correspondence to: María Luisa Zúñiga, PhD, Assistant Professor, Director of Program Evaluation, UCSD Division of Community Pediatrics, University of California, San Diego, 9500 Gilman Drive, Mail Code 0927, La Jolla, CA 92093 (E-mail: mzuniga@ucsd.edu).

[Haworth co-indexing entry note]: "Exploring Care Access Issues for Mexican-Origin Latinos Living with HIV in the San Diego/Tijuana Border Region." Zúñiga, María Luisa et al. Co-published simultaneously in *Journal of HIV/AIDS & Social Services* (The Haworth Press, Inc.) Vol. 5, No. 2, 2006, pp. 37-54; and: *Outreach and Care Approaches to HIV/AIDS Along the US-Mexico Border* (ed: Herman Curiel, and Helen Land) The Haworth Press, Inc., 2006, pp. 37-54. Single or multiple copies of this article are available for a fee from The Haworth Document Delivery Service [1-800-HAWORTH, 9:00 a.m. - 5:00 p.m. (EST). E-mail address: docdelivery@haworthpress.com].

Available online at http://jhaso.haworthpress.com
© 2006 by The Haworth Press, Inc. All rights reserved.
doi:10.1300/J187v05n02_05

SUMMARY. Health access issues and dynamics of health access for Latinos living with HIV on the U.S.-Mexico border have not been well-characterized. Health service utilization and related issues unique to seropositive HIV Latino populations were explored and findings are presented from two focus groups with Mexican women and men living with HIV in the San Diego/Tijuana U.S.-Mexico border. Cross-cutting border issues (same as Trans-border issues) included lack of continuity in HIV treatment options in Mexico, provider and social stigma of AIDS patients in Mexico, and fears of crossing the border to the U.S. for appointments. Findings indicate a need for coordinated bi-national efforts at HIV/AIDS research and services for border region inhabitants. doi:10.1300/J187v05n02_05 *[Article copies available for a fee from The Haworth Document Delivery Service: 1-800-HAWORTH. E-mail address: <docdelivery@haworthpress.com> Website: <http://www.HaworthPress.com> © 2006 by The Haworth Press, Inc. All rights reserved.]*

KEYWORDS. Latinos, HIV, AIDS, U.S.-Mexico border, health access

INTRODUCTION

The uniqueness of the U.S.-Mexico border's transnational, social, economic, and cultural matrix warrants improved understanding of health access dynamics for Latinos living with HIV in this region. Previous HIV studies have not documented health access issues for HIV seropositive Mexican-origin Latinos who live on the border and cross it on a regular basis, a trans-border population. Preliminary findings are presented from two focus groups conducted with Mexican women and men living with HIV in the San Diego/Tijuana U.S.-Mexico border region. Information from this small qualitative pilot study is intended to inform research questions for future studies to better understand and meet the needs of Latino populations living with HIV in the U.S.-Mexico border region.

The Current Study

The purpose of the current pilot study was to explore barriers and facilitators to service utilization on the part of seropositive Latino men and Latina women living in the U.S.-Mexico border region. Exploratory research questions included: (1) Which factors inhibit and which facilitate the use of needed health and related services on the part of HIV seropositive Latinos living in the U.S.-Mexico border region? (2) Do HIV seropositive Latina women and Latino men experience different barriers and facilitators to access services? and (3) Are there access to care barriers and facilitators specific to the U.S.-Mexico border region? In February 2001, two focus groups were held at a community-based health clinic in San Ysidro, California. This non-profit clinic is located two miles from Tijuana, Baja California, Mexico, and provides HIV/AIDS services for a predominantly Mexican-origin trans-border population.

BACKGROUND

The United States-Mexico (U.S.-Mexico) border region represents a unique environment for health-seeking behavior of persons who live and work in this region, particularly for those who have access to health services on both sides of the border. Many of the U.S. counties along the U.S.-Mexico border are designated as medically underserved areas (Health Resources and Services Administration [HRSA], 2004), which may contribute to trans-border health-care choices. The uniqueness of the border environment is also observed in patterns and burden of infectious and chronic diseases, which are oftentimes different than patterns and burden within the interior of the U.S. (HRSA; Doyle & Byran, 2000). HIV/AIDS is an infectious disease that has been identified as one of 20 priority health objectives in the U.S.-Mexico Border Health Commission's Healthy Border 2010 Program (U.S.-Mexico Border Health Commission, 2003; Notzon, 2001). Regional data from San Diego County, which borders Tijuana, Baja California, Mexico, indicates that Mexican-origin Latinos in the border region account for a disproportionately high number of AIDS cases. In San Diego County, the recent AIDS case rate for Latino males was 69.8 per 100,000 (April 2000 to March 2002), second only to the African American male case rate of 110 per 100,000 and appreciably higher than the case rate for White males, at 33.5 per 100,000 (San Diego County Office of AIDS Coordination, 2002). For Latinas in San Diego, the AIDS case rate was 8.8 per 100,000, versus 23.2 for African American females and 3.3 for White females (San Diego County Office of AIDS Coordination).

Differences in health indicators and health-care utilization have been documented for Mexican-origin Latino populations living along the

U.S.-Mexico border as compared to Latinos living in other regions (Besser et al., 2001; Doyle & Bryan, 2000; Guendelman & Jasis, 1992; Guendelman & Jasis, 1990). In a survey of Tijuana residents regarding health-care utilization practices, Guendelman and Jasis (1990) observed that predictors of health-care use in the U.S. included insurance coverage, transportation, older age and being male. Research efforts have only recently begun to assess health utilization and health disparities in HIV/AIDS along the U.S.-Mexico border (Ruiz, 2002), including health-care issues unique to Latinos living with HIV. Preliminary data indicate that HIV seropositive Mexican-origin Latinos receiving HIV medical services in San Diego, California, also routinely cross the border for health care or medications in Mexico (Southern California Border HIV/AIDS Project, 2005). Health-care consumer choices appear to be access-based as well as economically driven (Southern California Border HIV/AIDS Project).

Home to about 10 million persons, the U.S.-Mexico border extends 1,864 miles east to west (Texas to California) and 62 miles north and south of the international boundary. San Diego has the busiest border crossing in the world, with 41.8 million northbound border crossing registered in 2000 (U.S. Customs Service, 2001). U.S. Census 2000 figures indicate that counties with the highest proportions of Latinos were along the southwestern border of the U.S. (U.S. Census Bureau, 2001).

Published information regarding the expressed needs and problems encountered by HIV seropositive and AIDS-affected Latinos living in the border region is limited. California Office of AIDS recently conducted an unpublished study of high-risk predominantly Mexican men who have sex with men (MSM) living in Tijuana, Baja California, and San Diego, California (Ruiz, 2002). High levels of HIV infection were found in both groups, with seropositivity levels of 19% (47/240) for Tijuana MSMs and 35% (44/125) for San Diego MSMs. Nearly half of the Tijuana sample and three-quarters of the San Diego sample reported sex with partners from across the border, and men at both sites reported engaging in high rates of unprotected anal and vaginal sex with multiple male and female sex partners (Ruiz). Because unique identification and reporting of HIV cases began only recently in California ([CA] Office of AIDS, 2002), future HIV seroprevalence studies will better elucidate true HIV prevalence in Latino populations.

METHODOLOGY

Conceptual Framework

According to Strauss and Corbin (1990), the concept of grounded theory can be used to approach general and basic interest in a topic area when there is no specific hypothesis to test or theory to prove. This approach to the current small exploratory study seemed appropriate in view of the paucity of literature on the topic area. Thus, the idea was to facilitate discussion/conversation with participants by using a semi-structured focus group format to elicit general commentary about their lives as HIV seropositive Mexican men and women living in the U.S.-Mexico border region (e.g., through open-ended questions), as well as specific stories and information about access to HIV/AIDS services (e.g., through specific questions and prompts about factors that have facilitated and inhibited their access). The overarching goal of this approach is to begin to generate basic information about an under-researched topic area for future development of more specific research questions and methods.

Setting

San Ysidro Health Center (SYHC) is a community-based non-profit health center located two miles from the U.S.-Mexico border that provides comprehensive primary care services to residents of San Diego County's South Bay Region. SYHC is the only provider of HIV/AIDS services in the South Bay and offers a continuum of culturally competent, client-centered medical and social support services for people who are infected or affected by HIV/AIDS. SYHC is a federally qualified health center (FQHC). As such, the health center receives approximately $2.2 million annually to subsidize the delivery of health-care services to uninsured individuals and families through SYHC's sliding fee scale (SFS) program. Uninsured patients pay for health-care services and prescription medicines based on their ability to pay. Ability to pay is determined by total household income and number of people living in the household. All HIV/AIDS services are available in both English and Spanish. In order to receive HIV services at SYHC, HIV seropositive clinic patients, including the participants in this study, must fulfill residency requirements, have proof of diagnosis, and a valid identification. Actual country of residence, however, may be on either side of the border.

Participants

Participants were part of a broader five-year multi-site border initiative (Southern California Border HIV/AIDS Project) that is being carried out to assess health promotion and continuity of care issues for HIV seropositive persons living in the U.S.-Mexico border region. The focus group participants were a convenience sample of HIV seropositive clients who received care at the clinic. Clients were invited to participate by case managers and volunteered through a sign-up sheet posted at the agency reception area. This study was reviewed and approved by the University of California, San Diego Human Research Protection Program. A voluntary consent statement was read to focus group participants and their permission to tape the session was obtained prior to initiating the discussion. A $25 food voucher incentive was provided to volunteer participants. Nine HIV positive Mexican women participated in the women's group, and nine HIV positive predominantly gay Mexican men that have sex with men (MSM) participated in the men's group. Mean age for participants in the women's group was 40 years (range 27 to 51 years). Seven of the nine women had not completed high school. All women had gone to school in Mexico and two of them had received education in the U.S. and in Mexico. Average family household size was 3.7 persons, with number of children ranging from 0 to 3. All of the women self-identified as heterosexual and were either married, widowed or lived with an opposite sex partner. The mean age for the men's group was 41 years (range 33 to 46 years). Five of the participants had not completed high school. Average family household size was 2.5 persons; none of the men self-reported as married and no children were reported in the Latino men's group. All of the male participants in this study self-identified as gay or bisexual.

Procedures

A series of open-ended questions and follow-up prompts was constructed by the second author to conduct semi-structured focus group discussions focusing on four well-known dimensions of human and social service utilization:

1. *Availability of services*, which refers to the existence of services;
2. *Accessibility of services*, which refers to service convenience or affordability;

3. *Acceptability*, which refers to how congruent services are with client expectations (cultural);
4. *Accountability*, which refers to service system responsiveness to clients.

Focus groups were conducted by the second author, a researcher of HIV/AIDS with Mexican migrants, and by the fourth author, a trained project staff member. Both facilitators are bilingual (English/Spanish), bicultural Latinos/as. Groups were conducted in Spanish and lasted an average of two hours each. Focus group sessions were tape recorded, transcribed in Spanish, and coded and analyzed.

Analysis of Data

A content analysis plan was developed to analyze focus groups' comments and dialogue. Content analysis is a technique to categorize textual information (e.g., focus group transcripts) to determine frequencies within predetermined categories (Denzin & Lincoln, 1994; Van der Veer Martens, 2001; Webb & Kevern, 2000). As an initial assessment of coding reliability, coders were asked to independently review and manually code 5% of the text for the women's focus group (~722 words) in order to establish inter-rater reliability. This test resulted in 92% agreement between raters. Coding for the men's focus group was carried out by one of the two above coders. Loss of coding staff resulted in only one of the coders being able to complete coding for the men's focus group, however, coding results for both groups underwent detailed review by the project's lead investigator, who is also bilingual.

Primary coding themes in Spanish-language text were entered into, and analyzed separately for each focus group, using the Qualitative Solutions and Research (QSR), Non-numerical Unstructured Data Indexing Searching and Theorizing (NUD*IST) software package (Qualitative Solutions and Research, 1997). Once analysis was conducted, findings were translated from Spanish into English by the lead author of this study.

Coding Scheme

The four dimensions of health and social services were used as coding schemes to analyze study participant comments. Definitions of these coding themes are provided in Table 1. As themes were identified in the text, coders noted whether the theme included a barrier or facilita-

TABLE 1. Coding Themes Used in Focus Group Content Analysis

	Theme	Criteria
Theme 1	Availability of Services	• Are services available in the geographic area?
Theme 2	Accessibility to Services External service factors	• If services are available, are they accessible to the client? For example, client transportation, money or insurance to pay for the service, information written at an appropriate reading level for clients, etc.
Theme 3	Acceptability of Services External service factors Internal client/cultural factors	• Are services acceptable to clients? Do services meet client cultural and social expectations and needs? For example, language needs, cultural sensitivity, etc. Does the client feel comfortable using the service? Internal/personal issues of service acceptability include client's personal/internal stigmas (e.g., homophobia or ashamed to seek AIDS services, etc.)
Theme 4	Accountability of Services to the Clients/Community	• Do services have mechanisms whereby consumers can participate in service decision-making or provide feedback on services they receive? For example, community advisory boards, suggestion boxes, etc.

tor to service use. Coders further identified whether service issues were internal (e.g., client perceived, homophobia) or external (e.g. interpreter services were poor). This subcoding allowed for improved understanding of client interaction with the health-care delivery system. In an effort to discern those barriers specific to the San Diego/Tijuana, U.S.-Mexico border service region, where possible, distinction was made between barriers identified within and outside the San Diego border region.

RESULTS

Latina Women's Focus Group

Theme 1: Availability of Services

Lack of childcare was a predominant concern expressed by Latinas. They discussed needing childcare for doctor visits and other activities.

One respondent stated, ". . . the only way they can help us is to have someone care for the children." Latinas perceived that a lack of child care was an issue for both men and women caregivers. One woman also felt that there are more services for adults than for children, noting lack of access to a clinical trial for her child.

Other problems with service availability included lack of access to a psychologist, limited clinic hours, too few HIV/AIDS support groups, lack of continuity with clinicians, and concerns with seeking care at locations where these women could be identified and stigmatized by others. Some women expressed dissatisfaction with services for women because they perceived that HIV/AIDS services are geared toward homosexual men, namely gay identified MSMs. This issue was raised three times during the focus group.

Latina participants felt that the availability of HIV/AIDS support groups and clinical research trials, that included medical services for children, were important facilitators for meeting their health and family needs. One woman's HIV was diagnosed through her prenatal care and she was offered an opportunity to enroll in a clinical trial. Her child was born HIV-negative.

Theme 2: Accessibility of Services

A frequently expressed personal/cultural barrier pertained to husbands/male partners. Latina women discussed fear of a partner's response to their seeking HIV/AIDS services and the experience of husbands discounting the value of support group participation. Participation in a support group, as perceived by the husband of one participant, meant that the woman's participation in other family activities (e.g., going out to dinner) was compromised. Issues of being submissive to male partners were also raised in the discussion of barriers. One woman stated that not until her husband died did she start to participate in support groups: "If I had my husband, I wouldn't be attending meetings, and possibly I would not be here." The irony of these statements is striking considering that nearly all participants indicated that they had been infected by their husbands/male partners as has been substantiated in the literature as the major risk factor for Mexican women (Cohn & Clark, 2003; Organista, Balls Organista, Garcia de Alba G., Castillo Moran, & Ureta Carrillo, 1997; Salgado de Snyer, Diaz Perez, & Maldonado, 1996). Access recommendations included improved outreach to other infected women with messages to take health information and become better informed. One participant told of an experience in which, once she became engaged in services, her partner followed suit and now both are participating in therapy.

Theme 3: Acceptability of Services

Perceived excessive waiting time for appointments in some service settings was a barrier and area of concern for Latina participants: "I feel out of place. I see everyone go in and out to see the doctor and I'm sitting there for hours and hours, until I start to cry, I get depressed and leave." Other concerns included language barriers, dissatisfaction with switching providers without prior notification from the service provider, and dissatisfaction with services viewed as geared towards male homosexuals. One respondent stated: "I feel that there it's more for gay men, gay persons." Another stated: "I feel like they [service providers] don't pay the attention that I deserve. . . . I feel as if I were a plant on a chair, and everyone comes and goes, especially homosexuals."

Many responses were linked to stigma and respondents referred to a fear of being stigmatized by the surrounding community: "What if they see you in a place where only infected people go, then they'll know you're infected." Participants mentioned that a lack of knowledge of HIV/AIDS in the Latino community also affects them: "Within the Hispanic community their not knowing anything about AIDS is worse . . . that is, they are still afraid that if you touch them, or if they drink from your soda." Fear of the participant's families being stigmatized if anyone knew of the participant's HIV status was also discussed. Other responses included cultural issues in reference to approaching physicians, such as not voicing concerns because of deference to doctors and the perception that the doctor is always right. Despite these observations on cultural barriers, it is important to note that female participants expressed overall satisfaction with their current clinical providers and case managers at the clinic where the focus groups were conducted.

Theme 4: Accountability of Services

Latina participants felt comfortable providing feedback about clinic services either in person or confidentially, through a suggestion box at the clinic. Latinas mentioned a perceived lack of accountability in terms of child-care needs that had not been adequately addressed after they had voiced this issue during local AIDS planning council meetings.

Latino Men's Focus Group

Theme 1: Availability of Services

Overall, Latino men felt that adequate services were available to them at the clinic where focus groups was conducted. Lack of dental services was mentioned among barriers in San Diego, and lack of medication and services outside San Diego were also mentioned. Informational brochures were considered helpful in letting clients know about services.

Theme 2: Accessibility of Services

Public transportation and distance to services was a major barrier mentioned in the Latino men's focus group: ". . . because we have to go to San Diego, we would always miss appointments because of the distance and having to take the trolley." Another barrier identified was not being able to receive vitamins or medications for secondary complications of HIV. One participant mentioned that those without a social security number face barriers in accessing services.

Theme 3: Acceptability of Services

Participants expressed satisfaction with clinic services received in San Diego. One barrier to acceptability of services was that instructions for prescriptions or some informational brochures are written in English: "I took the precaution of calling to ask what it meant [a prescription], and they told me it was for gargling . . . otherwise I would have been drinking three doses [of it], three times a day!"

Theme 4: Accountability of Services

Service accountability focused primarily on issues of the responsiveness of the university research community to its clinical trials participants. It was suggested that participants be assisted with access to housing or with an identification card that could be used if needed when crossing the border to participate in clinical trials.

Border-Specific Issues

Issues relevant to living in the U.S.-Mexico border region with HIV/AIDS were raised by both Latino male and female participants in ways that cut across the four primary coding/service themes. Border-specific issues included crossing the border; worries about going back and forth and not always being able to return for services in the United States. "The stress of crossing . . . it is a major issue, the idea that I get up and I know that I have an appointment and I'm nervous." Another participant stated: "It's a risk, if you cross you get services, if you're not permitted, you don't have services." Male participants acknowledge that HIV infection crosses the border with those who carry the disease: "A lot of infected people come [to Tijuana], and now we are exporting the infection once again to the United States." U.S. immigration policy on HIV varies by type of immigration status, and for some Mexican immigrants the threat of deportation may prevent them from seeking HIV testing or treatment for their disease (American Foundation for AIDS Research, 2001).

Although the need for linguistically appropriate services and resources is not uniquely a border issue, the demand for bilingual service providers, Spanish-language interpreters and service information, is particularly high along the border. Participants discussed a variety of language barriers, including not being able to obtain service information in Spanish, inadequate communication with providers, lengthy waits for interpreters, and poorly translated information.

Respondents from both groups voiced their experiences in Tijuana with not being able to obtain medications or continue with the same HIV medications, because providers had only different medications to offer. A female respondent stated, "Now if you are taking, for example . . . and you go to Tijuana they are going to prescribe what is available not what you need." One male respondent expressed fear of receiving services in Mexico and the negative treatment received from physicians in Mexico because of the perceived stigma of HIV/AIDS. Social stigma, both on the U.S. and Mexico side of the border, was commonplace in the focus group discussions. One respondent stated: ". . . for example in my *colonia* (neighborhood) in Tijuana where I was born and raised, I would not like it if they knew." Although not necessarily specific to the border region, easy access to homeopathic medication and alternative and complementary therapies are important health access and treatment considerations in the border region. Both groups mentioned access to homeopathic medicine and/or alternative therapy.

Participant Recommendations

Common recommendations from both groups included providing assistance to areas outside of San Diego, including the Tijuana region, where participants perceived a greater need for services. For San Diego, male participants recommended providing English classes as well as improvement in the quality of interpreter services and Spanish-language brochures.

Additional recommendations were to provide a form of identification to facilitate the border-crossing process as a means of participating in HIV/AIDS clinical trials. This type of arrangement is feasible, because it is currently available to some women and children who participate in HIV clinical trials through a special arrangement between the University of California, San Diego and the U.S. Immigration and Naturalization Services.

DISCUSSION

HIV and AIDS disproportionately affect Latinos and, in particular, Latinas represent a growing number of AIDS cases. Lags in diagnosis of HIV and access to treatment of HIV illness contribute to an over-representation of AIDS cases in communities of color, thus adding to disparities in health for minority populations.

Our results provide the following insights to the three guiding exploratory questions asked at the start of our study. Factors that inhibit or facilitate the use of needed health and related services on the part of HIV seropositive Latinos living in the U.S.-Mexico border region included issues such as transportation and child-care barriers. Although these issues are not unique to our population and are common to other HIV seropositive populations as found in periodic surveys conducted by the County of San Diego, we found that themes related to border issues or crossing from Mexico for services added a unique perspective to common issues identified by our participants. U.S. Policy on HIV seropositive immigrants, for example, contributes to anxiety felt by participants when they cross the border. Female participants also mentioned that their partners might negatively influence their participation in services such as support groups. Partner influence on participation in support groups may be an area for intervention through the patient's social worker. Probing for the level of partner influence and choice regarding health care or support group participation may provide the social worker with information on how to further enhance the patient's overall health. Women also expressed feelings of social stigma, another issue that impacts persons living with HIV on both sides of the border. To this effect, current Mexican government-sponsored Spanish-language radio media campaigns heard on both sides of the border are currently promoting awareness about the negative effects of social stigma of HIV seropositive persons.

Participants expressed overall satisfaction with care, mentioned by both the men's and women's groups. Given that satisfaction with care is an important indicator of health-care utilization (Aday, Anderson, & Flemming, 1980), this is a positive finding in our study. Differences between HIV seropositive Latina women and Latino men in terms of perceived barriers and facilitators to access services were found on the issue of childcare. Only the women participants raised concerns about issues related to childcare, a logical finding given that male participants did not report having children in their homes. This is a similar finding identified by HIV-infected women through surveys conducted by the San Diego County Office of AIDS Coordination (2002). We found as well that sensitivity to the environment of care where female participants perceived that clinics were more geared towards serving gay males, was gender-specific. Increased sensitivity to the environment of clinical practice settings that serve a variety of infected patients may include attention to gender and gay-related health promotion materials and routine feedback from patients.

Interestingly, both groups raised access to clinical trials as an area of concern. One woman mentioned it in the context of enrolling her child, and a male participant mentioned it in terms of having more support to cross the border to participate. The growing and dynamic nature of trans-border activity by Latinos living along the U.S.-Mexico border presents a unique set of circumstances and challenges for addressing HIV and AIDS that we are only beginning to understand. Access to care barriers and facilitators specific to the U.S.-Mexico border region were indicated by our participants. Participants stated that they had fear and anxiety about simply crossing the border (the usual procedure of going through U.S. Customs) from Mexico to the U.S. for care. Apprehension about crossing the border while in possession of one's HIV medications is a source of anxiety for some patients due to fear of losing one's permit to cross the border. Non-U.S. citizens who are HIV seropositive are denied entry into the U.S. without a special waiver (Goldberg, 1998; Webber, 2005)

Many HIV seropositive patients regularly cross the border and seek health care on both sides of the border. Data on trans-border behavior from participants in the broader multi-site initiative support our qualitative findings in this study. Data on 116 HIV seropositive border residents in our San Diego-based border HIV study show that 64% of respondents (74 out of 116 persons) reported 12 or more round trips to Mexico in the last year (range 12 to 365 roundtrips) (Southern California Border HIV/AIDS Project, 2002). Respondents in this broader study also report accessing health services in Mexico within the last year, with about half reporting having obtained medications in Mexico (Southern California Border HIV/AIDS Project). Although Latinos living with HIV along the U.S.-Mexico Border appear to face similar barriers to accessing health care as other U.S. Latinos, the dynamics of being a largely trans-border population add a new challenging dimension to health-care access, where communication between providers, health administrators and policymakers, on both sides of the border, becomes an increasingly important goal yet to be fulfilled.

This was a pilot study using a qualitative approach to explore care access in an HIV serpositive Mexican-origin, border-dwelling population about whom little has been published. Limitations to this study are many and include small group size, limited number of groups, and limited ability to understand individual experiences outside a group context. As a pilot study, we are limited in our ability to generalize findings to other border populations. Larger sample sizes will be needed in order to determine the reliability of findings. Participant perceptions of access issues may differ from those of the broader patient population of patients living with HIV served in our study clinic. Our participant sample of convenience was based on a small number of Latinas and Latinos living with HIV/AIDS who are recipients of services at a community clinic less than one mile north of the U.S.-Mexico border. Experiences of trans-border Latinos living with HIV from this clinic may differ from experiences of clients in other clinics in the San Diego-Tijuana region and elsewhere along the U.S.-Mexico border. These limitations should be addressed in future studies.

Future research questions raised as a result of this study include:

1. What are contributing factors to health disparities in accessing services for border populations living with HIV?
2. What are contributing factors to health disparities in clinical trials participation for Latinos living with HIV?
3. How does engaging Latinas living with HIV into care affect their participation in support groups or other forms of support?
4. How does improved access to care for Latinas living with HIV impact the care participation of their HIV-affected partners?

5. What are the patterns of bi-national utilization of alternative or complementary therapies for Latino border populations and which alternative and/or complementary therapies are most commonly used?

Addressing these research questions would allow for more effective outreach to and care for border inhabitants living with HIV as well as benefit other HIV-affected Latinos in the U.S.

Our exploratory work is a first step towards assessing the breadth and scope of health service issues for Latinos living with HIV along the U.S.-Mexico border. We feel that issues of immigration status will present an additional burden of inclusion into health-care options for these persons living with HIV. As the health research community confronts low representation of minority persons in clinical research studies, new options for inclusion of border or undocumented populations should also be explored. Trans-border health-care access activity also merits further strategy development and further investigation with the goal being improvement in the health of border-dwelling Latinos living with HIV.

AUTHOR NOTE

The current study is part of a broader five-year border HIV/AIDS demonstration project funded in 2000 by the U.S. Department of Health and Human Services, Health Resources and Services Administration (HRSA), HIV/AIDS Bureau, Ryan White Care Act Special Projects of National Significance Program. This project was also partially supported by Grant Number P60 MD00220, from the San Diego EXPORT Center, National Center of Minority Health and Health Disparities, National Institutes of Health, and Grant Number 1K01 MH072353-02 from the National Institutes of Mental Health. Its contents are solely the responsibility of the authors and do not necessarily represent the official views of the National Institutes of Health.

REFERENCES

Aday, L. A., Anderson, R., & Flemming, G. V. (1980). *Health care in the U.S.: Equitable for whom?* Beverly Hills, CA: Sage Publications, Inc.
American Foundation for AIDS Research (2001). People with HIV face U.S. immigration ban. Retrieved August 6, 2002 from http://www.amfar.org/cgi-bin/iowa/news/record.html?record=70

Besser, R. E., Pakiz, B., Schulte, J. M., Alvarado, S., Zell, E. R., Kenyon, T. A. et al. (2001). Risk factors for positive Mantou Tuberculin Skin Tests in children in San Diego, California: Evidence for boosting and possible foodborne transmission. *Pediatrics, 108*(2), 305-310.

California Office of AIDS (2002). HIV reporting regulations became effective July 1, 2002. California Department of Health and Human Services. Retrieved November 2002, from http://www.dhs.cahwnet.gov/aids/HIVReporting/HIVReporting.htm.

Cohn, S. E., & Clark, R. A. (2003). Sexually transmitted diseases, HIV, and AIDS in women. *Medical Clinics of North America, 87*(5):971-95.

Denzin, N. K., & Lincoln, Y. S. (Eds.) (1994). *Handbook of qualitative research.* Thousand Oaks, CA: Sage Publications.

Doyle, T. J., & Bryan, R. T. (2000). Infectious disease morbidity in the U.S. region bordering Mexico, 1990-1998. *Journal of Infectious Diseases, 182*, 1503-10.

Goldberg, S. B. (1998). Immigration issues and travel restrictions. The Body: The Complete HIV/AIDS Resource. Retrieved July 21, 2005 from http://www.thebody.com/encyclo/immigration.html.

Guendelman, S., & Jasis, M. (1992). Giving birth across the border: The San Diego-Tijuana connection. *Social Science and Medicine, 34*(4), 419-25.

Guendelman, S., & Jasis, M. (1990). Measuring Tijuana residents' choice of Mexican or U.S. health care services. *Public Health Reports, 105*(6), 575-583.

Health Resources and Services Administration (2004). U.S.-Mexico Border Health. Bureau of Primary Health Care, U.S. Department of Health and Human Services.

Notzon, S. (2001). Healthy people 2010: History and health measures. National Center for Health Statistics, Centers for Disease Control and Prevention. Retrieved June 10, 2004 from http://www.borderhealth.org/files/res_68.pdf

Organista, K. C., Balls Organista, P., Garcia de Alba G., J. E., Castillo Moran, M. A., & Ureta Carrillo, M. E. (1997). Survey of condom-related beliefs, behaviors, and perceived social norms in Mexican migrant laborers. *Journal of Community Health, 22*(3), 185-198.

Qualitative Solutions and Research, Non-Numerical Unstructured Data Indexing, Searching and Theorizing User Guide (1997) (QSR NUD*IST) *User Guide* (1997). Thousand Oaks, CA: Sage Publications Inc.

Ruiz, J. D. (2002). *HIV prevalence, risk behaviors and access to care among young Latino MSM in San Diego, California and Tijuana, Mexico.* (Data presentation dated March 2002). Epidemiology Branch, Office of AIDS, California Department of Health Services. Sacramento: California Office of AIDS, CA Department of Health Services.

Salgado de Snyder, V. N., Diaz Perez, M. J., & Maldonado, M. (1996). AIDS: Risk behaviors among rural Mexican women married to migrant workers in the United States. *AIDS Education and Prevention, 8*(2), 134-142.

San Diego County Office of AIDS Coordination (2002). *San Diego County AIDS cases: Regional proportion of cases by five year cohort*, Reported through March 31, 2002. San Diego: San Diego County Office of AIDS Coordination.

Southern California Border HIV/AIDS Project (2005). (Unpublished data). University of California, San Diego, San Diego, CA.

Strauss, A. L., & Corbin, J. M. (1990). *Basics of qualitative research: Grounded theory procedures and techniques.* Newbury Park, CA: Sage Publications.

U.S. Census Bureau; U.S. Department of Commerce, Economics and Statistics Administration, (2001). *The Hispanic population; Census 2000 brief,* Guzmán, B.

United States Customs Service (2001). *Fiscal Year 2000 port crossings* (California border with Mexico).

United States-Mexico Border Health Commission (2003). Healthy border 2010: An agenda for improving health on the United States-Mexico border. Retrieved June 10, 2004 from http://www.borderhealth.org/files/res_63.pdf

Van der Veer Martens, B. (2001) Research techniques for information management (Science and Technology Center Course: IST 501). Retrieved June 10, 2004 from http://web.syr.edu/~bvmarten. Syracuse, NY: Syracuse University.

Webb, C., & Kevern, J. (2000). Focus groups as a research method: A critique of some aspects of their use in nursing research. *Journal of Advanced Nursing, 33*(6), 798-805.

Webber, D. W. (2005). Summary of U.S. law on entry of noncitizens with HIV. AIDSandtheLaw.com–An HIV/AIDS law & policy resource. Retrieved on December 19, 2005 at http://www.aidsandthelaw.com/issues/entry%20to%20US.htm.

doi:10.1300/J187v05n02_05

HIV/AIDS Outreach
in Southern New Mexico:
From Design to Implementation

Michelle Valverde, PhD
Jennifer Felderman-Taylor, MA

SUMMARY. This paper describes the outreach component of the New Mexico Border Health Initiative (NMBHI), one of five Special Projects of National Significance funded in 2000 along the United States/Mexico border by the Health Resources and Services Administration. The initial intent of the NMBHI was to utilize the traditional *promotor* model of natural helpers within the informal support systems in the communities in which they physically live for the purpose of increasing utilization

Michelle Valverde, PhD, is Adjunct Assistant Professor at the Department of Sociology and Anthropology, New Mexico State University.

Jennifer Felderman-Taylor, MA, is Research Analyst II for the County of Los Angeles Department of Health Services Office of AIDS Programs and Policy.

Address correspondence to: Michelle Valverde, PhD, Department of Sociology and Anthropology, MSC 3BV, New Mexico State University, P.O. Box 30001, Las Cruces, NM 88003 (E-mail: mvalverde@zianet.com).

The authors would like to thank David Barney, PhD, and Betty Duran, MSW, MPH, from the School of Social Work at New Mexico State University, Herman Curiel, PhD, at the University of Oklahoma, and the collaborating partners.

This publication is supported by Grant Number 5 H97 HA 00186-02 from the Health Resources and Services Administration (HRSA) Special Project of National Significance (SPNS) Program. This publication's contents are solely the responsibility of the authors and do not necessarily represent the official view of HRSA or the SPNS Program.

[Haworth co-indexing entry note]: "HIV/AIDS Outreach in Southern New Mexico: From Design to Implementation." Valverde, Michelle, and Jennifer Felderman-Taylor. Co-published simultaneously in *Journal of HIV/AIDS & Social Services* (The Haworth Press, Inc.) Vol. 5, No. 2, 2006, pp. 55-71; and: *Outreach and Care Approaches to HIV/AIDS Along the US-Mexico Border* (ed: Herman Curiel, and Helen Land) The Haworth Press, Inc., 2006, pp. 55-71. Single or multiple copies of this article are available for a fee from The Haworth Document Delivery Service [1-800-HAWORTH, 9:00 a.m. - 5:00 p.m. (EST). E-mail address: docdelivery@haworthpress.com].

Available online at http://jhaso.haworthpress.com
© 2006 by The Haworth Press, Inc. All rights reserved.
doi:10.1300/J187v05n02_06

of HIV/AIDS prevention services. What evolved instead was more closely aligned with traditional street outreach, whereby peers were utilized to engage and inform potential clients about HIV prevention, provide HIV testing and link HIV-affected persons to medical services. Programmatic elements, implications for practice, and recommendations for program coordinators are presented in the paper. doi:10.1300/J187v05n02_06 *[Article copies available for a fee from The Haworth Document Delivery Service: 1-800-HAWORTH. E-mail address: <docdelivery@haworthpress.com> Website: <http://www.HaworthPress.com> © 2006 by The Haworth Press, Inc. All rights reserved.]*

KEYWORDS. U.S./Mexico border, HIV/AIDS, outreach, testing, demonstration, HIV outreach worker, promotor

INTRODUCTION

The New Mexico Border Health Initiative (NMBHI) at *Camino de Vida* ([CdV], Road to Life) Center for HIV Services in *Las Cruces*, New Mexico (NM) was a five-year Special Project of National Significance (SPNS) funded from 2000 to 2005 by the Health Resources and Services Administration (HRSA), HIV/AIDS Bureau. The NMBHI was one of five funded research and demonstration sites providing HIV/ AIDS services along the United States/Mexico border. Data collection for evaluation purposes began in March 2001 and continued through December 2004.

Prior to the implementation of the NMBHI in 2000, the focus at CdV was on providing case management services to persons living with HIV/AIDS in southern New Mexico. This included but was not limited to the coordination of medical care and supportive services. With the development of the NMBHI, the scope of services provided at CdV expanded to include outreach prevention with the explicit goals of (1) increasing HIV testing, (2) raising the awareness of individuals at risk about the importance of knowing their HIV status and early detection, and (3) enrolling individuals who test seropositive for HIV into medical care early in the cycle of the disease.

National data illustrate that many individuals with HIV get tested late in the progression of the disease. Of those who do get tested, many never receive their test results (Centers for Disease Control [CDC], April 2003). Data collected from May 2000 to February 2003 at 16 HIV testing and counseling sites across the country, revealed significant differences between early and late testers. In contrast to early testers, late testers were more likely to have lower levels of formal education, be exposed to HIV through heterosexual contact, and be Hispanic or Black (CDC, June 2003).

One detrimental result of late testing is delayed HIV diagnosis and subsequent access to medical and social services. Late testing also results in missed opportunities for preventing the spread of HIV given that the time period between initial HIV infection and diagnosis is when infected individuals can unknowingly transmit HIV to others. Thus, both the CDC and HRSA stress the importance of designing outreach programs that focus on specific populations at risk for late HIV testing.

As one such population at risk, Hispanics are not only overrepresented among those who test late for HIV, they are also overrepresented among new U.S. AIDS cases. Hispanics comprised 12 percent of the U.S. population in the year 2000, yet they represented 19 percent of the total number of new AIDS cases reported (CDC, 2002). It is important to point out that while race and ethnicity by themselves are not risk factors for HIV infection, social and economic elements such as higher rates of poverty and limited access to health care increase the risk for infection among Hispanics (CDC, 2002). Other dimensions related to race/ethnicity, language, gender, and sexual behavior also contribute to increased HIV/AIDS risk (Diaz, 1998).

In the counties where CdV services were offered, Hispanics represent approximately 60 percent of the general population (U.S. Census Bureau, 2000). The proportion of Hispanic HIV clients at CdV has increased, up from 47 percent in 1997 to approximately 57 percent in 2004. In addition to an increasing proportion of Hispanic clients at CdV, many continue to enter care late in the progression of the disease. It is highly probable that the well-documented barriers to accessing health care in the region, such as the lack of medical insurance, high rates of poverty and unemployment, and a shortage of health-care providers (Health Resources and Services Administration, 1998) are contributing to the problem of late entry. With 316,000 people living in an area of 32,000 square miles (U.S. Census Bureau), long distances between communities and, thus, medical providers, may also be a contributing factor.

FROM PROMOTORES *TO HEALTH OUTREACH WORKERS*

As mentioned above, the primary goals of the NMBHI outreach component were to increase HIV testing, to raise the awareness of individuals at risk about the importance of knowing their status and the benefits of early detection, and to enroll individuals who test positive for HIV into medical care early. The three primary groups targeted by the NMBHI were (1) men who have sex with men (MSM), (2) intravenous drug users (IDU), and (3) women at risk for HIV infection. Added emphasis was placed on reaching Hispanics given AIDS' disproportionate impact on their communities, and their historical lack of access to health care in general.

To accomplish these goals, the initial intent of the NMBHI plan was to utilize traditional *"promotores,"* most often defined as "natural helpers" who are members of informal support systems within their communities (Earp & Flax, 1999; Eng, Parker, & Harlan, 1997) in which they physically live. A number of other terms are found in the literature to describe the concept of *promotores.* These include lay health workers, indigenous lay workers, lay health advisors, community health workers, community health advisors, *consejeras,* health aides, navigators, and outreach workers (Candelaria, Campbell, Lyons, Elder, & Villaseñor, 1998; Earp & Flax; Eng, Parker, & Harlan). Generally these individuals are local leaders who are both concerned about their communities and familiar with their peers (Altpeter, Earp, Bishop, & Eng, 1999; Candelaria et al.). According to the literature, *promotores* are often volunteers who do not receive monetary compensation for their work (Eng, Parker, & Harlan; Thomas, Eng, Clark, Robinson, & Blumenthal, 1998).

Most frequently *promotores* in the U.S. are aides to professional staff in promoting preventative health care in areas such as prenatal care, childhood immunizations, breast and cervical cancer screening, hypertension reduction, smoking cessation, and the use of primary health care (Earp & Flax, 1999). Some lay health advisors serve as "outreach arms" of formal organizations to link community members to professional care providers (Eng, Parker, & Harlan., 1997; Salber, 1979) while others strive to support positive behavior change (Candelaria et al., 1998; Thomas, Earp, & Eng, 2000).

The NMBHI contracted interested individuals professionally and/or personally familiar with HIV/AIDS to conduct outreach to at-risk populations beyond their respective geographic home communities. In contrast to this, *promotores,* as described in the literature, most often live in the communities they serve. Another important role distinction is that most of the NMBHI outreach workers held full-time professional positions in addition to being contracted to work for CdV.

Given the salient differences between traditional *promotores* and the NMBHI model, it became clear by the end of the first year of the program that the original intent had not materialized. This realization prompted discussions between the local evaluator, SPNS program staff, and the outreach workers themselves, resulting in the title change from *promotores* to health outreach workers (HOWs) in year two of the project. Despite the fact that both *promotores* and street outreach workers strive to (1) reach groups who do not normally access traditional western health-care systems, (2) refer historically underserved individuals to social and health services, and (3) deliver health information and materials in the field wherever the contact may occur (Altpeter et al., 1999; Valentine & Wright-deAgureo, 1996), the differences were inescapable.

What had evolved instead was more closely aligned with traditional street outreach, whereby peers were utilized to test, support, and engage potential clients. The use of peers was an essential feature of the NMBHI, which is typical of most street outreach programs (Anderson et al., 1996). As such, each NMBHI HOW, although not living in the targeted community, shared a familiarity with either intravenous drug use, men who have sex with men, and/or women at risk for HIV.

For example, the two HOWs hired to target intravenous drug users, one female and one male, were former IDUs themselves. One was the director of the methadone maintenance facility in southern New Mexico and the other was a "recovering" active member in a local support group. The HOW hired to primarily target women at risk had worked with underserved populations for more than 10 years, most recently as a full-time nurse at the methadone maintenance clinic. Because she lived in Mexico for 12 years and was Spanish proficient, she was able to reach out to Spanish-speaking women.

Like HOWs working with IDUs, HOWs assigned to do outreach work with the MSM population shared the same sexual orientation. One HOW was a dual resident of *Ciudad Juarez,* Mexico and *El Paso*, Texas. He had prior work experience at CdV as a peer advocate and was a volunteer with an AIDS service organization in *Ciudad Juarez.* As an open bilingual and bicultural Hispanic gay male, he was able to relate more easily to persons and institutions on both sides of the U.S.-Mexico border. A second bicultural Hispanic HOW who was native to New Mexico (NM) also worked with MSMs and had previous volunteer experience with the agency. A gay male living with HIV/AIDS joined the outreach team in fiscal year four in addition to functioning as a peer advocate. His perspective in terms of living with the disease was both powerful and pivotal for the program. As a peer advocate, he provided transportation, education, and emotional support to CdV clients and helped coordinate the support group activities. He went on to provide prevention case management and group level interventions and support within the agency as a full-time prevention specialist.

In addition to the differences between traditional *promotores* and the NMBHI HOWs, the realities of testing individuals for HIV and collecting data in the field made the NMBHI outreach model unique. The vast majority of *promotor* projects in southern NM are family-centered and focus on topics such as maternal child health, diabetes, immunizations, asthma, and toxic pesticides. *Promotor* projects that do focus on HIV/AIDS have only recently gone beyond offering prevention education to include testing and counseling. The location of contact was another distinguishing factor of the NMBHI HOWs since they interacted with individuals not just in homes and community centers, but also in homeless and domestic violence shelters, halfway houses, bars, and on the street.

One facet of the HOW model that facilitated client access to HIV prevention services in the rural communities was partnering with other *promotor* projects. Partnerships were established with a *promotora* project focused on HIV prevention education with Families and Youth, Inc., *Mujeres Unidas en Accion Contra el SIDA* (*MUACES*–Women United in Action Against AIDS), and with the *promotores* working with a CdV contract provider, the Ben Archer Health Center. Collaborative outreach activities were conducted in the southern NM communities of Hatch, Anthony, Chaparral, Sunland Park, and Anapra as a result of these partnerships. Collaborations with other *promotor* projects in the area not only increased referrals for HIV testing but also served to establish linkages with health-care gatekeepers in several smaller communities. The introduction of HIV testing in the field by the NMBHI resulted in a network for shared training opportunities and capacity building in rural areas, which are benefits that will last beyond the funding period of the NMBHI.

PROGRAMMATIC AREAS

To increase the identification and HIV testing of MSM, IDU, and women at risk for HIV infection, and increase the linkage of individuals who test positive for HIV with services early in the cycle of the disease, the project team established four broad program areas: (1) *recruitment and training of the HOWs*, (2) *HIV testing the targeted high-risk individuals*, (3) *raising HIV risk awareness of the targeted individuals*, and (4) *linking newly diagnosed individuals into HIV primary care*.

Recruitment and Training of the HOWs

The first program element consisted of the recruitment of the HOWs, which was accomplished by tapping into existing networks of individuals who were personally and/or professionally familiar with HIV/AIDS. Although job announcements were placed in the local newspaper, word of mouth advertising through community leaders and collaborating agencies proved to be most effective in recruiting candidates for the HOW positions. Immediately after being hired, the HOWs received a two-day training offered through the New Mexico Department of Health (NMDOH) in order to become certified in HIV testing and counseling.

Based on the client-centered "Fundamentals of HIV Prevention Counseling" curriculum from the CDC (U.S. Department of Health and Human Services, 1999), every HOW learned how to implement the six-step protocol in the field: (1) Introduce and orient the individual to the session, (2) identify the individual's personal risk behaviors and circumstances, (3) identify safer goal behaviors that the client can adopt, (4) develop a risk reduction action plan, (5) make referrals, and (6) bring closure to the session. In order to meet the requirements for the NMBHI, the CdV HOWs, in collaboration with the evaluation team, added two steps, data collection and the follow-up meeting, to the standard six steps of testing and counseling (see Table 1). This protocol is discussed in greater detail below.

Before conducting outreach alone in the field, each HOW was also required to shadow an experienced tester and to receive field safety and data collection training. Quarterly trainings on a variety of topics identified by the HOWs, the program coordinator, and/or the evaluation team, were found to be critical in meeting the educational needs of the HOWs in providing skilled services and remaining motivated. This supports earlier findings from other successful outreach programs around the country about the importance of ongoing staff training (Cheney & Merwin, 1996; Greenberg et al., 1998; Kalinoski & Rothermel, 1995). Weekly outreach staff meetings facilitated by the program coordinator allowed each HOW to give an update of activities and recent challenges. The entire team learned from each other by lending support and problem solving.

HIV Testing the Targeted Individuals

In relationship to the second programmatic area, contacting and testing the targeted number and type of individuals at risk, the HOWs

TABLE 1. New Mexico Border Health Initiative: Eight-Step Protocol

1) Introduction

    A) Describe project and role of HOW

    B) Assess interest in participating

    C) Assess knowledge of HIV/AIDS

    D) Provide basic HIV/AIDS education

2) Describe Procedures

    A) OraSure test; returning the results

    B) Data collection

3) Complete Paperwork

    A) Consent form

    B) DOH bubblesheet

4) Collect Data/Provide Counseling

    A) Modules 5, 6, and D

    B) Assess risks and risk behaviors

    C) Identify safer goal behaviors that the individual can adopt

    D) Develop a risk-reduction action plan

5) Administer OraSure Test

    A) Explain how the OraSure test works

    B) Follow the procedures

6) Complete Self-administered Questionnaire

    A) Provide instructions

    B) Assist individuals if needed

7) Close Session

    A) Thank individuals for participation

    B) Respond to questions

    C) Make referrals and provide support

    D) Review follow-up plan to return results

8) Complete Follow-up

    A) Return test results; complete paperwork

    B) Provide incentives

focused on Doña Ana County (DAC), the most heavily populated county in the southern part of the state, an area which is also contiguous to Texas and Mexico. Due to the amount of time needed to participate in the study, participants received a $20.00 gift certificate redeemable at a local department/grocery store. Through a cooperative agreement with the NMDOH's Infectious Disease Bureau, OraSure HIV tests were provided free of cost whether the individuals agreed to participate in the study or not. As recommended by the U.S. Department of Health and Human Services (1999), individuals were contacted and/or tested in a number of environments to ensure that HIV counseling, testing, and referral services were provided in outreach settings to high-risk individuals who might not have access to clinical settings.

In the southernmost part of the same county, door-to-door outreach was conducted and group outreach occurred via *platicas* (talks) with between one and as many as eight participants in a single session. *Platicas* usually occurred during the day and involved mostly women. Such *platicas* were hosted by individuals who were referred to the HOWs by *promotoras* from *MUACES* as mentioned above. In addition to these efforts, individual contacts and tests were done in homes in another community based on word-of-mouth referrals. These educational groups usually occurred in the evenings and on weekends depending on the schedule of the HOW. In Las Cruces, the largest city in the county, contacts and tests were conducted at a halfway house and at homeless and domestic violence shelters. Contacts and tests were also conducted at public locations where drug activity and sex work occur. Most often these contacts were made at night, both during the week and on weekends in order to better reach these target populations.

While individual level interventions were conducted at all of these locations, educational group games were offered at select sites where interest existed. The educational group games facilitated the introduction of HIV basic education and the hierarchy of HIV risks, which allowed for open discussion and the development of prevention and harm reduction strategies.

Pre- and post-test counseling information about the transmission and prevention of HIV/AIDS was provided to all of the volunteer participants tested. As part of the testing and counseling process, specific information was collected on a standard form required by the NMDOH Infectious Disease Bureau. If the individual agreed to participate in the SPNS study and signed the necessary consent form, additional information was then gathered. Such information included basic demographics and behavioral HIV risk factors, which were collected through an interview process (Health Resources and Services Administration, 2001). Participants' self-perceived levels of awareness about the importance of early detection and knowing one's HIV status as well as HIV prevention knowledge were collected through a self-administered questionnaire developed and piloted locally. These data were helpful for the program and evaluation staff in monitoring whether the target populations were being reached. The data were also used, as described in the next section, to evaluate the impact of the contact with the HOW.

The typical session lasted an average of 30 minutes. Although the program coordinator encouraged the HOWs to follow the eight-step protocol in a linear fashion, individual variations in styles and the need to be client-centered may have contributed to variations in the length of the interviews.

Such flexibility resulted in each HOW developing a somewhat unique way of completing the process, while making sure to cover the required steps. For instance, one of the HOWs preferred to have the consent form signed (step 3A) right after assessing the individual's interest in participating in the study (step 1B), while another HOW preferred to assess for HIV risk behaviors (step 4B) before assessing HIV/AIDS knowledge (step 1C).

The turn around time for the OraSure test results from the state laboratory was approximately two weeks. Well-established testing and counseling sites and the agencies' routine hours available in the targeted communities helped ensure test results were returned and available in a timely manner. The volunteer participants could choose to be tested anonymously or confidentially. It was not surprising that many participants chose confidentiality given the availability of the HOW model, which provided a trusting relationship with a peer who knew the system and was familiar with HIV/AIDS and risk behaviors. The HOWs also provided business cards with their mobile phone numbers and the agency's toll-free number. The main advantage of being tested confidentially is that it expedited the post-test counseling process.

Demographics of Participants Reached via Outreach

The majority of the CdV participants in this study who were tested for HIV (n = 1,021) between March 2001 and December 2004 were male (56 percent, n = 572), Hispanic (67 percent, n = 684), and had a high-school diploma or less (82 percent, n = 837). Poverty was a factor for the majority of these participants as 67 percent reported household income of $10,000 or less (n = 684). Table 2 captures the risk categories by gender (note that the risk categories are not mutually exclusive). These risk categories reflect the NMBHI program priorities and are in no way intended to serve as an epidemiological description of the agency service area.

Raising the Awareness of the Targeted Individuals

The third area of emphasis of the NMBHI HOW component was raising the awareness of the high-risk individuals who were tested about their perception of the importance of knowing their HIV status and the benefits of early detection. In order to determine the importance of knowing their HIV status, a post-retrospective self-administered questionnaire was administered utilizing a four-point Likert scale of (1) "not at all important," (2) "not important," (3) "somewhat important," and (4) "very important."

Initial results suggest 96 percent of the participants (n = 877) provided answers acknowledging the "importance of knowing [their] HIV status" after contact with their HOW, whereas only 60 percent responded this way prior to meeting their HOW.

TABLE 2. Risk Demographics

Risk Category	Males (n = 572)		Females (n = 449)		Total (n = 1,021)	
	#	Percent	#	Percent	#	Percent
Multiple partners	403	71%	222	49%	625	61%
Other drugs	353	62%	156	35%	509	50%
Alcohol	351	60%	164	37%	515	50%
Incarceration	300	52%	120	27%	420	41%
Homeless	201	35%	107	24%	308	30%
IDU	138	24%	61	14%	199	20%
Sex partner IDU	115	20%	89	20%	204	20%
MSM	172	30%	N/A	N/A	172	17%
Forced sex	36	6%	105	23%	141	14%
Sex work	37	7%	55	12%	92	9%
Mental health	34	6%	17	4%	51	5%

A dichotomous question regarding whether participants (n = 767) knew about the benefits of early detection for HIV was answered affirmatively by 88 percent of the respondents after contact with their HOW, whereas 61 percent responded this way prior to contact with their HOW.

Linking Newly Diagnosed Individuals with HIV Primary Care

The fourth and final element of the CdV health initiative was to link newly diagnosed individuals with HIV primary care. This was facilitated through a partnership with the NMDOH's early intervention nurse who helped expedite the enrollment process into services. A standard procedure in the HIV testing and counseling protocol is for all individuals with positive OraSure test results to have a confirmatory HIV blood test completed. This test is usually collected by the early intervention nurse or another designated staff member at the NMDOH.

In addition to the support of NMDOH staff, the personal relationship established with the HOW during the process of completing the initial and confirmatory HIV tests was a key element in helping to link newly diagnosed individuals with care. During slightly more than 3.5 years of outreach through the NMBHI, 2,126 individuals were contacted by the HOWs. Of these, 1,021 were tested for HIV and participated in the study with approximately 79 percent receiving their test results. Six of the individuals who received an HIV test through outreach tested positive. Of these six, one was lost to follow-up in the first year of the project, three enrolled at CdV, and two enrolled at an agency in a larger city nearby.

The percent of positives identified through the NMBHI outreach component were as follows: 2002–.4 percent (1 tested positive out of 282), 2003–0 percent (0 tested positive out of 382), and 2004–1.1 percent (4 tested positive out of 366). Data from 2001 are not included because outreach started that year in late March. The NMBHI outreach data can be compared to the statewide "field" data, which includes NMBHI data, for the same calendar years. The percent of positives identified for the entire state was .4 percent in 2002, .8 percent in 2003, and .8 percent in 2004 (New Mexico Department of Health, 2002, 2003, and 2004). Given the lower prevalence of living HIV/AIDS cases in southwest NM at 94.1 per 100,000 compared to the state at large with 152.1 per 100,000 (HIV/AIDS Epidemiology Program, 2005), the NMBHI outreach effort appears to have been consistent with state data in two out of the three years examined.

The majority of HIV cases identified through outreach testing in the project were due to the relationship with the HOW, who also served as a peer advocate. In a separate example of the effects of this program, a former participant who tested negative for HIV with one of the HOWs, tested positive at a later date during a hospital stay. This HIV-affected person phoned the HOW for support in entering medical care. The individual began receiving the HIV care needed within one month after receiving the HIV diagnosis.

DISCUSSION AND IMPLICATIONS FOR PRACTICE

Although the original plan of the CdV NMBHI was to utilize the grassroots traditional public health, community-based *promotor* outreach model to conduct HIV/AIDS testing and counseling in the field, the strategy that emerged after one year more closely resembled traditional street outreach. The most salient differences that set the NMBHI HOWs apart from traditional *promotores* were that the HOWs worked outside their respective geographic communities and they were compensated monetarily. However, they shared similar ties of current or past sexual and/or drug-risk behaviors with the targeted individuals. Furthermore, all but one of the HOWs held professional positions in addition to conducting HIV outreach. Although it was found that the original *promotor* model did not materialize, it was determined that HIV/AIDS outreach programs, utilizing a client-centered model based on what works at the local level, must be able to adapt.

In developing the model in southern NM, some of the greatest challenges were related to the state's large rural areas and the complexity of doing outreach in the field (i.e., collecting data, executing HIV counseling and education, and the handling of specimens for HIV testing). Other challenges stemmed from the geographic expansiveness of rural NM and reaching the outlying communities. Sheer travel time and the difficulty in establishing routine hours in distant communities posed barriers to implementing the program outside DAC. The negative stigma associated with HIV/AIDS is yet another factor that made it difficult to reach individuals most at risk for contracting HIV. A strong indicator of the negative stigma is that three of the top six barriers for clients before entering HIV care were that "others would find out they were HIV positive," "others would think badly of them," and "others would think they were gay or lesbian" (based on survey results from 95 CdV clients who participated in SPNS).

Some limitations of this study involved the management and completion of data collection instruments and consent forms, and the recruitment and retention of HOWs. Although outstanding candidates surfaced through word of mouth advertising, Latina applicants were consistently not available.

Some changes in the program were based upon client feedback that resulted from the model being client-centered. The program continued to evolve even in the latter years of the initiative. The addition of peer advocates to the outreach team is one example of a modification that helped to increase the number of positives identified. In the southern part of DAC, *MUACES*, a partner agency, was able to begin providing HIV testing and counseling in the field in 2004, in part, due to the NMBHI collaboration and the capacity that had been built in prior years. HIV testing and counseling were also offered by the Ben Archer *promotoras* in the northern part of the county beginning the same year.

Readers interested in developing aspects of this outreach model for their own communities might benefit from the recommendations developed from this NMBHI project. Suggestions are offered in Table 3 regarding the issues of recruitment and training of HOWs, ideas for learning about HIV testing and raising the awareness of the targeted individuals, and ideas about ways to link newly diagnosed seropositive individuals with the HIV primary care systems.

The formal HIV testing and counseling guidelines served as the foundation for the NMBHI HOW model. Along with the encouragement and support of the staff coordinator, each HOW applied these guidelines to create his or her own unique approach. HOWs' life experiences, their knowledge of the medical and social service systems, and familiarity with HIV helped them tremendously in connecting with individuals who have historically been disconnected from health and social services. By providing HIV testing and counseling, sharing information, collecting data, and linking individuals into care, the HOWs made all participants more aware of HIV and the benefits of HIV testing, and more able to identify HIV risk; they linked to medical services those participants who were identified as HIV-affected. These interventions made a positive difference for the health care of residents in southern New Mexico.

TABLE 3. Lessons Learned

Recruitment and Training of HOWs

Use formal and informal avenues (word-of-mouth) to recruit HOWs; recruitment of peers is essential

Develop an initial and ongoing evaluation process to assess HOW knowledge, skills, and attitudes

Review the steps of HIV testing and counseling periodically and provide a checklist for the HOWs

Provide initial and ongoing trainings to keep the HOWs motivated, informed, and supported

Testing the Targeted Individuals

Modify the outreach strategies if the objectives are not being achieved; this may involve recruiting new HOWs

Partner with other agencies and *promotores* to expand geographic coverage and build capacity

Establish consistent hours of testing at community-based sites to increase return rates

Utilize different approaches to reach the MSM population; a focus on men's health issues is one strategy

Build in a quality assurance process to help support the HOWs in consistently following the protocol

Raising the Awareness of the Targeted Individuals

Identify the gatekeepers in the target communities and subpopulations and build relationships with them

Remain flexible and encourage the HOWs to adapt as needed

Promote the use of interactive educational approaches such as games when possible

Linking Newly Diagnosed Individuals into HIV Primary Care

Utilize a variety of strategies to return the test results to individuals; this is a critical step in the linkage process

Support the HOWs in providing transportation to potential clients

Provide translation services whenever needed

Provide training and a resource guide for the HOWs about community services

Ensure that the linkage process is client centered and as supportive as possible

REFERENCES

Altpeter, M., Earp, J. L., Bishop, C., & Eng, E. (1999). Lay health advisor activity levels: Definitions from the field. *Education and Behavior, 26*(4), 495-512.

Anderson, J. E., Cheney, R., Clatts, M., Faruque, S., Kipke, M., & Long, A. et al. (1996). HIV risk behavior, street outreach, and condom use in eight high-risk populations. *AIDS Education and Prevention, 8*(3), 191-204.

Candelaria, J., Campbell, N., Lyons, G., Elder, J. P., & Villaseñor, A. (1998). Strategies for health education: Community-based methods. In S. Loue (Ed.), *Handbook of Immigrant Health*. New York: Plenum Press.

Centers for Disease Control (2002). Fact sheet. HIV/AIDS among Hispanics in the United States. Retrieved on July 22, 2004 at <http://www.cdc.gov/hiv/pubs/hispanic.html>

Centers for Disease Control (April 2003). Advancing HIV prevention: New strategies for a changing epidemic–United States, 2003. *Morbidity and Mortality Weekly Report, 52*(15), 1-2.

Centers for Disease Control (June 2003). Late versus early testing of HIV–16 sites, United States, 2000-2003. *Morbidity and Mortality Weekly Report, 52*(25), 581-586.

Cheney, R., & Merwin, A. (1996). Integrating a theoretical framework with street outreach services: Issues for successful training. *Public Health Reports, 111*, 83-89.

Diaz, R. (1998). *Latino gay men and HIV: Culture, sexuality, and risk behavior*. New York: Routledge.

Earp, J. L., & Flax, V. L. (1999). What lay health advisors do. *Cancer Practice, 7*(1), 16-21.

Eng, E., Parker, E., & Harlan, C. (1997). Lay health advisor intervention strategies: A continuum from a natural helping to paraprofessional helping. *Education and Behavior, 24*(4), 413-416.

Greenberg, J. B., MacGowan, R., Neumann, M., Long, A., Cheney, R., Fernando, D. et al. (1998). Linking injection drug users to medical services: Role of street outreach referrals. *Health and Social Work, 23*(4), 298-310.

Health Resources and Services Administration (1998). *Assuring a healthy future along the U.S.-Mexico Border. A HRSA priority*. U.S. Department of Health and Human Services.

Health Resources and Services Administration, Special Project National Significance, United States/Mexico Border Health Initiative (2001). *Questionnaires: Risk factors*. Norman, OK: University of Oklahoma.

HIV/AIDS Epidemiology Program (2005). HIV/AIDS in New Mexico fact sheet. New Mexico Department of Health. Retrieved on August 30, 2005 at <http://www.health.state.nm.us/hiv-aids.html>

Kalinoski, J., & Rothermel, C. (Dec. 1994/Jan. 1995). Lessons from the street: Outreach to inner city youth. *SIECUS Report, 23*(2), 14-20.

New Mexico Department of Health (2002, 2003, and 2004). *Tests and positive tests by demographics, site type, test type, and previous test*. Public Health Division, Infectious Disease Bureau.

Salber, E. J. (1979). The lay advisor as a community health resource. *Journal of Health Politics, Policy and Law, 3*(4), 469-478.

Thomas, J. C., Earp, J., & Eng, E. (2000). Evaluation and lessons learned from a lay health advisor programme to prevent sexually transmitted diseases. *International Journal of STD & AIDS, 11*, 812-818.

Thomas, J. C., Eng, E., Clark, M., Robinson, J., & Blumenthal, C. (1998). Lay health advisors: Sexually transmitted disease prevention through community involvement. *American Journal of Public Health, 88*(8), 1252-1253.

U.S. Census Bureau; State and County Quick Facts (2000); Retrieved on June 10, 2004 at <http://quickfacts.census.gov/qfd/states/35000.html>

United States Department of Health and Human Services, Public Health Service (1999). *Fundamentals of HIV prevention counseling, Trainer's guide.*

Valentine, J., & Wright-deAgureo, L. (1996). Defining the components of street outreach for HIV prevention: The contact and the encounter. *Public Health Reports, 111*, 69-76.

doi:10.1300/J187v05n02_06

A Training Program Designed to Increase the Capacity of Community Health Centers Along the United States-Texas-Mexico Border to Treat HIV Infection

Gary I. Sinclair, MD
Yolanda Cantu, MPH, DrPH Candidate

SUMMARY. Resource poor regions, medically underserved by most measures, face particularly difficult challenges with regard to maintaining an adequate pool of HIV-competent physicians, physician assistants, and nurse practitioners. This paper describes a project designed to expand HIV care capacity in a resource poor community along the United States-Texas-Mexico border, utilizing existing community health centers. The authors describe their experiences in implementing and evalu-

Gary I. Sinclair, MD, is Assistant Professor of Medicine at The University of Texas Southwestern Medical Center at Dallas.

Yolanda Cantu, MPH, DrPH Candidate, is Assistant Professor of Pediatrics at The University of Texas Health Science Center, San Antonio.

Address correspondence to: Gary I. Sinclair, The University of Texas Southwestern Medical Center, 5323 Harry Hines Boulevard, Dallas, TX 75390 (E-mail: gary.sinclair@utsouthwestern.edu).

This work was supported by grant #H97HA00187 from the Health Resources Service Administration's Special Projects of National Significance (HRSA/SPNS). The publication's contents are solely the responsibility of the authors and do not necessarily represent the official view of HRSA or the SPNS program.

[Haworth co-indexing entry note]: "A Training Program Designed to Increase the Capacity of Community Health Centers Along the United States-Texas-Mexico Border to Treat HIV Infection." Sinclair, Gary I., and Yolanda Cantu. Co-published simultaneously in *Journal of HIV/AIDS & Social Services* (The Haworth Press, Inc.) Vol. 5, No. 2, 2006, pp. 73-88; and: *Outreach and Care Approaches to HIV/AIDS Along the US-Mexico Border* (ed: Herman Curiel, and Helen Land) The Haworth Press, Inc., 2006, pp. 73-88. Single or multiple copies of this article are available for a fee from The Haworth Document Delivery Service [1-800-HAWORTH, 9:00 a.m. - 5:00 p.m. (EST). E-mail address: docdelivery@haworthpress.com].

Available online at http://jhaso.haworthpress.com
© 2006 by The Haworth Press, Inc. All rights reserved.
doi:10.1300/J187v05n02_07

ating an AIDS Education and Training Center (AETC) physician training program. doi:10.1300/J187v05n02_07 *[Article copies available for a fee from The Haworth Document Delivery Service: 1-800-HAWORTH. E-mail address: <docdelivery@haworthpress.com> Website: <http://www.HaworthPress.com> © 2006 by The Haworth Press, Inc. All rights reserved.]*

KEYWORDS. Resource poor regions, United States-Mexico Border, HIV primary care, physician training, community health centers, increasing system capacity

INTRODUCTION

The shortage of competent providers of medical care in resource poor regions of the United States is known to be an impediment to equal access to care, particularly for minorities and other vulnerable populations (Blumenthal, 2003; Cooper, Getzen, McKee, & Laud, 2002). Resource poor regions are medically underserved by most measures (Hargraves, Cunningham, & Hughes, 2001; Kingston & Smith, 1997; Lewin Group, 1998), and face particularly difficult challenges in maintaining an adequate pool of HIV competent physicians, physician assistants, and nurse practitioners (McKinney, 2002).

Ample evidence links physician knowledge, skill, and experience (Bach, Calhoun, & Bennett, 1999; Brosgart et al., 1999; Curtis, ,Paauw Wenrich, Carline, & Ramsey, 1995; DeRiemer, Daley, & Reingold, 1999; Gerbert, Moe, & Saag, 2001; Heath, Bally, Yip, O'Shaughnessy, & Hogg, 1997; Kitihata et al., 1996; Kitihata, Van Rompaey, & Dillingham, 2003; Kitihata, Van Rompaey, & Shields, 2000; Landon, Moe, & Saag, 2003; Landon, Wilson, & Wenger, 2002; Stone, Mansourati, Poses, & Mayer, 2001; Willard, Liljestrand, Goldschmidt, & Grumbach, 1999) and health-care system experience (Laine et al., 1998; Markson, Houchens, Fanning, & Turner, 1998) with outcomes in HIV therapy. Furthermore, federally funded training programs have been shown to have positive effects on HIV provider knowledge and practice patterns (Huba, Panter, & Melchior, 2000; Lalonde, Uldall, & Huba, 2002).

Little work, however, has been done to evaluate the ability of specific training models and programs to bridge the gap between existing expertise, and the increasing demand for HIV treatment providers in resource poor settings (McKinney, 2002).

From 2000-2004, the authors of this paper participated in a research and demonstration project designed to expand the capacity of the resource poor south Texas-Mexico border public health care system to provide HIV primary care. This aim was in part operationalized through the development, implementation and evaluation of an AIDS Education and Training Center Program designed to increase the number of HIV-competent physicians in the project target sites.

In this article, we will discuss the implications that our experiences in implementing this training program may have for physicians, administrators, and other health-care professionals who seek to expand capacity to treat the HIV-infected.

DESCRIPTION OF THE SOUTH TEXAS BORDER PROJECT

Background

The project was primarily implemented in the three-county region along the Texas-Mexico border which is commonly referred to as the Lower Rio Grande Valley (Hidalgo, Willacy, and Cameron Counties). At project start, these three counties had reported 336 cases of HIV and 1,143 cases of AIDS (Texas HIV/STD Surveillance Report, 2002). The area had experienced a 28% population growth between 1990 and 2000 (from 661,370 estimated population in 1990 to 924,772 estimated population in 2000) (United States Census, 2000). The population of the region is overwhelmingly Hispanic and poor, with 34% of the region living at or below the poverty level, as compared to 15% for Texas as a whole (Texas Department of Health, 2000). As in most impoverished regions, the area is medically underserved. Direct care physicians number 1 per 920 residents, as compared to 1 per 620 residents for the state of Texas as a whole (Texas Department of Health, 2000).

In July of 2000, the Valley AIDS Council (VAC), the largest AIDS service organization (ASO) along the south Texas-Mexico border, received funding from the federal Ryan White Care Act for a research and demonstration project designed to improve access to HIV health care. Since its founding in 1988, VAC has provided medical care as part of its array of services exclusively for HIV-infected individuals. The agency had historically relied on one full-time physician to be the sole medical provider for all of its patients. However, at project start, the active caseload for this one physician had risen to more than 500 patients, with as many as 100 new patients projected per future year (Garcia, 2001). In addition, physician turnover issues had at times left VAC with no physician. As a potential solution to this limited and fragile HIV care capacity problem, VAC sought to partner with an existing network of federally qualified Community Health Centers (CHCs) in the lower Rio Grande Valley (LRGV) communities of Brownsville and McAllen/Pharr, and in the neighboring south Texas community of Eagle Pass. In the proposed model, VAC would supply HIV expertise, HIV medications, support services, and technical assistance with regard to the administration of the Ryan White Care Act funds, while the CHCs would provide a more secure supply of physicians.

Early project implementation activities with the CHCs, however, revealed a major barrier. Though eager and willing to help in the HIV epidemic, the CHC physicians did not feel they had an adequate knowledge base to competently manage HIV infection. Prior to the project, the CHC physicians promptly referred all known HIV-infected patients to the VAC for all medical needs. Already overburdened with the existing epidemics of diabetes, hypertension, tuberculosis, depression, and obesity, the CHC physicians agreed to participate in the project, only if some form of HIV training program could be incorporated into their busy practices.

For assistance with the training component of system capacity development, the VAC turned to the Texas Oklahoma AIDS Education and Training Center (TOAETC), part of the national Ryan White Care Act mandated Aids Education and Training Center system. Historically, the TOAETC had focused most of its training efforts on major urban areas where HIV-infected individuals number in the tens of thousands. At the time of the project's start, the TOAETC had virtually no presence in the project sites, or in any of the small- to medium-sized communities in the region. For the border project to succeed, this traditional approach needed to change.

During the first months of the project, multiple meetings occurred between VAC, the three partner CHCs, an expert HIV specialist physician affiliated with the TOAETC who practices HIV medicine at a major academic medical center in Dallas, Texas, and project planner/evaluators. A training model was developed which addressed the concerns of the CHC physicians and met with their approval. We now refer to this model as the Continuous Mentored Patient Care or CMPC model.

We have previously described in detail the design and implementation of the CMPC model used during the first two years of the project (Sinclair, Cantu, Duggan, & Smith, 2003). What follows is an abbreviated description of the model and selected evaluation results from the first four years of the project.

Model Description

Project Partners. The project was a collaboration between the Valley AIDS Council of Harlingen, Texas, three Community Health Centers (CHCs) located in the south Texas-Mexico border region in the communities of Brownsville, McAllen/Pharr, and Eagle Pass, Texas, and the Texas-Oklahoma AIDS Education and Training Center (TOAETC). Project evaluation and planning support were provided by the University of Texas Health Science Center at San Antonio, whose evaluation team included individuals with experience in developing, implementing, and evaluating HIV health and human service programs and interventions. VAC and the evaluators had a long history of working together and had developed the original project proposal.

Physician Training Model. In the United States, physician training includes a four-year post baccalaureate doctoral studies course and a three- to seven-year period of residency. During residency, the trainee physician (the resident) is assigned primary responsibility for the health and well-being of a panel of patients, while training and supervision are provided "on the job" by a more experienced physician (the attending). We have come to call this kind of training Continuous Mentored Patient Care (CMPC). The project physicians repeatedly stated to us that "a residency-like training program" would be needed for them to become comfortable with HIV care. Based on this assertion, we developed our training model around the concept of CMPC.

Table 1 provides an overview of the roles of the training and trainee physicians in the Continuous Mentored Patient Care Model.

The CMPC, which would traditionally occur in a hospital setting where the trainees (residents) and the more experienced physicians (attendings) are co-located, was adapted into a model where the trainees (CHC physicians) are supported by a more experienced physician (the TOAETC HIV specialist physician) based at an institution hundreds of miles away. Adaptations which were necessary to deal with the distance included: site visits to south Texas by the TOAETC physician to deliver a limited number of didactic presentations about HIV; quarterly visits by the TOAETC physician to the CHC physicians' practices to see HIV patients together; distance consultation initiated by the CHC physicians via telephone, fax, e-mail, and paging. The TOAETC physician made a commitment to be available and responsive to the CHC physician "trainees" at all times.

To determine if the project could be sustained using only resources available in the south Texas border community, the HIV-experienced

TABLE 1. Physician Roles in the Continuous Mentored Patient Care

Role of the Trainee Physicians	Role of the Experienced Physician
(Resident Physician or CHC physician)	*(Attending Physician or TOAETC Specialist Physician)*
• Takes primary responsibility for panel of patients	• Makes himself/herself available to trainee physicians 24/7
• Performs initial evaluation	• Reviews initial evaluation of trainee*
• Formulates preliminary assessment of problem	• Reviews trainee assessment*
• Formulates preliminary plan of care	• Reviews trainee plan*
• Reviews assessment and plan with more experienced physician*	• "Spot checks" patients and evaluates whether or not progression is occurring as expected*
• Monitors patient and informs more experienced physician if things do not seem to be going according to plan*	• Provides continuous feedback, information, and suggests useful references for self-education to trainees
• Gains gradual independence and decreases reliance on more experienced physician as skill level increases	• Allows trainee gradually increasing independence and decreased supervision
• Begins to assume training responsibilities for less experienced physicians	

* Initially, these activities occur with regularity. As the trainee gains skills, reviews occur less regularly and with less stringency.

VAC physician, after participating in the model during the first two years, assumed the TOAETC physician role, while the TOAETC physician remained on board as a "back-up." Back-up activities included supporting the VAC physician with consults, and continued availability to CHC physicians as needed. The functional roles of the clinical staff involved in the project are outlined in Table 2.

Project Physicians Trained, AETC Consults, and Caseloads

During the course of the first four years of the project, five CHC physicians received HIV training through the CMPC model. For the purpose of confidentiality, we will refer to the CHCs as CHC-1, CHC-2, and CHC-3.

The initial physician at CHC-1 stayed with the project for two years and then left to take a job in another state. Due to physician staffing shortages, CHC-1 opted not to have another physician trained. The initial physician at CHC-2 stayed with the project for six months, and then

TABLE 2. Functional Roles of the Clinical Project Staff

Individual(s) in project	Year 1 and 2	Year 3 and 4
VAC Physician	• Observe process	• Take over role of the TOAETC physician
TOAETC HIV Specialist Physician ("the attending")	• Didactics for CHC physicians • Quarterly visits to CHCs • 24/7 distance consultation • Accept role of "experienced physician" in CMPC	• Served as backup consultant for the VAC physician
CHC Physicians ("the residents")	• Accept 2 new HIV patients into their practice/month • Accept role of "trainee physician" in CMPC	• Unchanged
CHC Nurses	• Coordinate HIV patients' medical care at the CHC with medication access and support services available through VAC	• Unchanged
VAC Nurses	• Work with CHC nurses to ensure that VAC medication access and support services would be available to CHC HIV patients	• Unchanged

also relocated out of state. The medical director at CHC-2 received training and covered the project for the next six months. Subsequently, a replacement was found for the initial project physician. This physician received training and has stayed with the project for three years. The initial physician at CHC-3 received training and has stayed with the project for four years.

The project physicians relied heavily on the TOAETC specialist physician for guidance as evidenced by frequent use of the consultation service into the fourth year of the project and beyond. Project physicians reported use of the VAC physician for consultation during the second half of the project. However, the specific numbers of consultations were not reliably recorded.

In spite of physician turnover, at the end of two years, the three CHCs demonstrated their capacity to provide local HIV primary care with their existing physician work force.

Table 3 summarizes physicians trained, consultation use, and patient caseloads at various times during the project. It should be noted that at project start, no HIV care was provided by any of the project CHCs.

TABLE 3. Project Physicians Trained, Consultations with TOAETC, and Patient Caseloads

Community Health Center	Number of Physicians Trained	Number of Physicians Currently Providing HIV Care	Number of Consults with TOAETC Physician	Physician HIV Patient Caseloads*	
				End of Year 2	End of Year 4
CHC-1	1	0		13**	NA
CHC-2	3	1	Years 1-2: 52	10	26
CHC-3	1	1	Years 3-4: 23	10	28

*All three CHC provided no specific HIV care at the start of the project.
**Peak number of patients served prior to CHC-1 withdrawal from the project during year 2.

EVALUATION OF THE MODEL

Evaluation Methodology

A qualitative evaluation of the model was conducted by the evaluation team. The evaluation team conducted six, 12, and 24-month open-ended interviews lasting approximately one hour with project physicians, nurses, and case managers/social workers during the first two years of the project. Annual interviews were conducted thereafter. Administrators and trainers were interviewed yearly throughout the project. The interviews explored and documented different aspects of participant experiences with the project model including satisfaction with the quality, amount and duration of training (including the consulting service), comfort levels with and attitudes towards HIV care provision, concerns and issues with model implementation and overall operation, as well as highlights and low points from their professional perspectives. Responses were recorded by the interviewers. Interviewer notes were transcribed and then analyzed. Responses to the questions were categorized by responder type into similar categories of responses and these were further synthesized into themes. Themes were frequently associated with issues or problems that the physicians and other project participants identified in the day-to-day project operations.

The project program evaluation protocol, methods and subject consents were reviewed and approved by the University of Texas Health Science Center at San Antonio Institutional Review Board responsible for human subjects protection oversight.

Themes

Prolonged Period of Educational Support

Three major themes repeatedly emerged. The first theme identified the need for a *prolonged period of educational support* for physicians from well-recognized, "24/7 available" HIV experts. Although satisfaction levels with the TOAETC specialist provider were high, the level of physician satisfaction dropped during years three and four of the project when the model could not maintain the same level of support when the VAC physician found himself to be too busy with patient care issues to provide the same level of service.

Also, although the project targeted physicians for training, nursing staff emphasized that the same level of discipline-specific training was needed for all professionals involved in the effort to increase system capacity to provide quality HIV care.

Physician Time and Compensation

The second theme raised the issues of physician *time and compensation*. CHC physicians repeatedly expressed frustration with the amount of time HIV care required from their already busy days. The physicians indicated that in order to provide quality HIV care, they had to "rob Peter to pay Paul" by taking time away from their non-HIV caseload. Vacations became an issue as other physicians in the CHCs felt unprepared to provide coverage for the clinic's HIV patients. CHC administrators were concerned about the discrepancy between the physicians' self-reported increased work load, and a drop in the total number of patients seen by the project physicians. The CHC physicians and administrators across all three sites pointed out that physician salary and compensation is strictly linked to numbers of patients seen per annum in the CHC system. The current system has no way of compensating for the extra time and effort required to receive HIV-related training, and to care for the more complicated HIV patients,

All CHC physicians and staff reported high levels of satisfaction about a training model that minimized the time burden by bringing HIV training and precepting on-site at the CHCs and the TOAETC physician's ready availability for distance consultation.

Patient Trust in the New System

The third theme identified the issue of *patient trust in the new system.* A major aim of VAC's partnership with the CHCs was to bring HIV primary care to the communities where the patients lived. However, both VAC and CHC staff reported reluctance on the part of the patients to seek medical care near their own homes. When surveyed, patients seemed to prefer the relative anonymity that a 40-minute drive to a neighboring community can provide.

Furthermore, project staff reported that patients tended to be suspicious of the new system of care. Some patients indicated that VAC was known throughout the lower Rio Grande Valley as "the best place to go for HIV." Other staff indicated that patients who had never experienced care at the VAC site were more likely to be satisfied with the care provided at the CHC.

Table 4 provides a sample of selected statements highlighting project participant concerns associated with the three themes identified in the interviews and associated with model implementation issues.

AN ILLUSTRATION OF THE MODEL IN ACTION

One of the project physicians received a call on a Sunday morning from the local hospital where he had admitting privileges. A critically ill patient recently diagnosed with AIDS had been admitted the night before. The physician who admitted the patient to the hospital confessed concern that he was ill-prepared to manage this patient's care, and asked the project physician for help. The project physician went to the hospital, evaluated the patient, called the TOAETC physician at his home in Dallas, and formulated a diagnostic and therapeutic plan.

The plan was not easy to implement. The patient required an intravenous medication that the hospital's pharmacy did not stock. The patient's family was shocked and frightened by the AIDS diagnosis, and unwilling to sign consent forms. The hospital staff expressed concern about the level of infection control precautions they needed to take when interacting with this patient. The laboratory staff refused to process some of the tests the physician had ordered as they had "never even heard of them." It was suggested that the patient be transferred to a tertiary care center immediately, at the hospital's expense.

The project physician felt that the patient would not survive a prolonged transport. He insisted that the patient be treated, and placed several calls to the hospital administration as well as to the chief of pharmacy.

Ultimately, an off-duty pharmacist drove six hours round trip, at his own expense, to pick up the needed medication. A social worker came

TABLE 4. Participant Themes on the Training Model

		Themes	
Project Staff	Prolonged Educational Support	Time and Compensation	Patient Trust
Physicians	"The medical school doctor is trained to be a mentor–I'm not."	"Mentoring takes time that I don't have."	"Patients don't trust the CHCs for HIV care."
	"The mentor needs to come to me. I don't have time to travel."	"HIV patients are more time consuming than others."	"I think the patients know I'm not an expert in HIV."
	"The mentor needs to be available 24/7."	"My income went down, my workload went up."	
	"Four years and I still need a mentor."	"Need to have coverage for my HIV patients when I leave town."	
	"The mentor should be a specialist from the Medical School."		
Nurses	"We need a nurse from the Nursing School to be our mentor."	"Need to hire more nurses specifically for HIV."	"Patients prefer to seek care away from home (privacy)."
	"Everyone in the clinic needs a mentor–not just the doctor."		"Patients know VAC is the best for HIV in the Valley."
			"Transportation not really a problem–despite no mass transit in the valley."
			"Patients worry about privacy–relatives get care here too."
CHC Administrators		"Physicians say they are working harder, but productivity measures fell."	"Other patients in the clinic think HIV patients are getting special treatment."
		"What do I do with the HIV patients if the trained physician goes on vacation or leaves?"	

83

forward, stated that she had a relative who had died of AIDS, and offered to counsel the family. The infection control nurse pulled the CDC literature regarding universal precautions and AIDS patients off of the Internet website, and educated the staff. The laboratory technician called a colleague from Dallas and learned how to appropriately process the requested samples.

The patient survived his acute illness, and was started on HIV medication. At last evaluation, his HIV was well-controlled and his prognosis deemed excellent.

CONCLUSIONS

Although many challenges were encountered, this project demonstrated that an AETC-driven physician education model can help Community Health Centers in smaller resource poor communities to develop the capacity to care for the HIV infected. We summarize below the training elements that seemed most critical to the success of our capacity expansion effort, the barriers that we encountered, and the challenges that remain for capacity expansion planners.

Training Elements Most Critical to Success: Prolonged Multi-Disciplinary Educational Support

Consistent with the conclusions of Gerbert et al. (2001), we found that physicians with minimal HIV expertise must be provided with respected HIV experts, who make themselves available for prolonged periods of time for consultation and educational support. The "medical tourist model," where a physician performs one or two site visits and "helps out" the local doctors in a superficial way will generally be met with distrust and hostility from the communities being asked to extend themselves in a capacity expansion effort. It is also unlikely to produce a competent HIV provider. Furthermore, the mentoring physicians must recognize the enormous time pressures that CHC physicians in smaller communities face, and make every effort to supply training in the most time-efficient way possible. Those who allocate funds for federal training programs may need to see physician training as a legitimate, reimbursable, and resource consuming activity. Physicians from academic medical centers, faced with their own pressures, are unlikely to engage in these kinds of training activities unless they receive monetary support in amounts sufficient to justify the time that it takes to do them well.

The work of Laine et al. (1998) and Markson et al. (1998) suggests that physician expertise accounts for only a portion of the competency equation. One can anticipate that once physicians are trained to provide HIV care, there will be a ripple effect throughout the systems in which they work. For capacity expansion efforts to be successful, Aids Service Organization directors, CHC administrators, and federally funded trainers need to have the capacity to provide education not only to the physicians, but to all those individuals necessary to support the endeavors that the physicians must integrate and coordinate. This includes all of the various disciplines and individuals who constitute the care team. While nurses, pharmacists, and dentists are critical, social workers, psychologists, pastoral counselors, clerical staff, laboratory personnel, family members, friends and, of course, the patient will have questions about HIV which require rapid answers.

Barriers: Time and Compensation

Federal policymakers need to recognize that HIV care is a labor intensive process that will tax the already overburdened organizations that will ultimately be asked to provide services to the growing numbers of HIV-infected individuals in resource poor regions. Capacity expansion efforts in resource poor communities, such as the border region, are unlikely to succeed unless creative ways are developed to recognize the increased demands being placed on all involved in HIV care, and to reimburse the individuals doing the work appropriately. As an example, the "one size fits all encounters" reimbursement system utilized by the Community Health Centers in determining physician compensation, is unlikely to provide for a fair and equitable allocation when a disease as complicated as HIV is in the mix. New ways of thinking about compensation (e.g., paying more for patient visits requiring more complicated medical decision-making) need to be adopted. Also, capacity expansion plans may have to include more than one physician in order to provide coverage when the primary HIV provider is not available.

Challenges: Patient Trust

Most importantly, the needs and reactions of patients must be taken into account when planning capacity expansion efforts. System change is a complex and gradual process that takes time even when well-executed. Users of the service system must be informed of changes and informed of the rationale for those changes. Although providing services in local communities seemed like a good idea at the outset of the project, our evaluation conformed to the findings of McKinney (2002) by revealing that concern for privacy continued to be a greater barrier to care in the project sites than transportation issues. The issue of patient trust has encouraged us to develop quality measures to ensure that the care provided at the CHCs is equivalent to the care being provided at the VAC. Future capacity expansion efforts should take into consideration the question of patient trust, and capacity expansion planners should build quality control measures into the initial plans.

As the AETC training models are exported into the international arena (see http://www.go2itech.org/), it is now more critical than ever to understand which elements of the AETC programs and policy have accounted for its successes (and failures) in the United States. While the evaluation of a project implemented in a limited geographic region cannot necessarily be generalized to other, even similar, regions, we expect that certain themes we have identified may prove to be valid across a wide variety of capacity expansion endeavors. The ability to identify universal themes and to develop useful evaluation instruments based on these themes, is critical to ensuring that future generations of capacity expanders will not have to relearn the painful lessons of the early days of the HIV epidemic in the United States.

REFERENCES

Bach, P. B., Calhoun, E. A., & Bennett, C. L. (1999). The relation between physician experience and patterns of care for patients with AIDS-related *pneumocystis carinii* pneumonia: Results from a survey of 1,500 physicians in the United States. *Chest, 199* (6), 1563-1569.

Blumenthal, D. (2003). Toil and trouble? Growing the physician supply. *Health Affairs, 22* (4), 85-87.

Brosgart, C. L., Mitchell, T. F., Coleman, R. L., Dyner, T., Stephenson, K. E., & Abrams, D. I. (1999). Clinical experience and choice of drug therapy for human immunodeficiency virus disease. *Clinical Infectious Diseases, 28*, 14-22.

Cooper, R. A., Getzen, T. E., McKee, H. J., & Laud, P. (2002). Economic and demographic trends signal an impending physician shortage. *Health Affairs, 21* (1), 140-153.

Curtis, J. R., Paauw, D. S., Wenrich, M. D., Carline, J. D., & Ramsey, P. G. (1995). Physicians' ability to provide initial primary care to an HIV-infected patient. *Archives of Internal Medicine, 155*, 1613-1618.

DeRiemer, K., Daley, C. L., & Reingold, A. L. (1999). Preventing tuberculosis among HIV-infected persons: A survey of physicians' knowledge and practices. *Prevention Medicine, 28*, 437-444.

Garcia, F. (2001), Developing HIV/AIDS health care in the United States-Mexico border [On- line]. Retrieved on September 14, 2002 from http://www.ou.edu/border/presentations/.

Gerbert, B., Moe, J. C., & Saag, M. S. (2001). Toward a definition of HIV expertise: A survey of experienced HIV physicians. *AIDS Patient Care and STDS, 15,* 321-330.

Hargraves, J. L., Cunningham, P. J., & Hughes, R. G. (2001). Racial and ethnic differences in access to medical care in managed care plans. *Health Services Research, 36* (5), 853-868.

Heath, K. V., Bally, G., Yip, B., O'Shaughnessy, M. V., & Hogg, R. S. (1997). HIV/AIDS caregiving physicians: Their experience and practice patterns. *International Journal of STD/AIDS, 8,* 570-575.

Huba, G. J., Panter, A. T., & Melchior, L. A. (2000). Effects of HIV/AIDS education and training on patient care and provider practices: A cross-cutting evaluation. *AIDS Education and Prevention, 12,* 93-112.

Kingston, R. S. & Smith, J. P. (1997). Socioeconomic status and racial and ethnic differences in functional status associated with chronic disease. *American Journal of Public Health, 87* (5), 805-810.

Kitihata, M. M., Koepsell, T. D., Deyo, R. A., Maxwell, C. L., Dodge, W. T., & Wagner, E. H. (1996). Physicians' experience with the acquired immunodeficiency syndrome as a factor in patients' survival. *New England Journal of Medicine, 334,* 701-706.

Kitihata, M. M., Van Rompaey, S. E., & Dillingham, P. W. (2003). Primary care delivery is associated with greater physician experience and improved survival among persons with AIDS. *Journal of General Internal Medicine, 18,* 95-103.

Kitihata, M. M., Van Rompaey, S. E., & Shields, A. W. (2000). Physician experience in the care of HIV-infected persons is associated with earlier adoption of new antiretroviral therapy. *Journal of the Acquired Immune Deficiency Syndrome, 24,* 106-114.

Laine, C., Markson, L. E., McKee, L. J., Hauck, W. W., Fanning, T. R., & Turner, B. J. (1998). The relationship of clinic experience with advanced HIV and survival of women with AIDS. *AIDS, 12,* 417-424.

Lalonde, B., Uldall, K. K., & Huba, G. J. (2002). Impact of HIV/AIDS education on health care provider practice: Results from nine grantees of the Special Projects of National Significance Program. *Evaluation in Health Professions, 25,* 302-320.

Landon, B. E., Wilson, I. B., & Cohn, S. E. (2003). Physician specialization and antiretroviral therapy for HIV: Adoption and use in a national probability sample of persons infected with HIV. *Journal of General Internal Medicine, 18,* 233-241.

Landon, B. E., Wilson, I. B., & Wenger, N. S. (2002). Speciality training and specialization among physicians who treat HIV/AIDS in the United States. *Journal of General Internal Medicine, 17,* 12-22.

Lewin Group (1998). The impact of the restructuring of the U.S. health care system on the physician workforce and vulnerable populations. *Report prepared for the Bureau of Health Professions, Division of Medicine.*

Markson, L. E., Houchens, R., Fanning, T. R., & Turner, B. J. (1998). Repeated emergency department use by HIV-infected persons: Effect of clinic accessibility and expertise in HIV care. *Journal of the Acquired Immune Deficiency Syndrome and Human Retrovirology, 17*, 35-41.

McKinney, M. M. (2002). Variations in rural AIDS epidemiology and service delivery models in the United States. *Journal of Rural Health, 18* (3), 455-466.

Sinclair, G. I., Cantu, Y., Duggan, S., & Smith, C. R. (2003). Training physicians to provide HIV medical care along the Texas-Mexico border: The Continuous Mentored Patient Care Model. *Texas Journal of Rural Health, 4*, 27-34.

Stone, V. E., Mansourati, F. F., Poses, R. M., & Mayer, K. H. (2001). Relationship of physician specialty and HIV/AIDS experience to choice of guideline-recommended antiretroviral therapy. *Journal of General Internal Medicine, 16*, 360-368.

Texas Department of Health (2000). Selected facts for Cameron County [Online]. Retrieved on September 14, 2002 from http://www.tdh.state.tx.us/dpa/cfs00/Camero00. pdf.

Texas Department of Health (2000). Selected facts for Hidalgo County [Online]. Retrieved on September 14, 2002 from http://www.tdh.state.tx.us/dpa/cfs00/Hidalg00. pdf.

Texas Department of Health (2000). Selected facts for Texas [Online]. Retrieved on September 14, 2002 from http://www.tdh.state.tx.us/dpa/cfs00/texas00.pdf .

Texas Department of Health (2000). Selected facts for Willacy County [Online]. Retrieved on September 14, 2002 from http://www.tdh.state.tx.us/dpa/cfs00/Willac00. pdf.

Texas HIV/STD Surveillance Report (2002) [Online]. Retrieved on September 14, 2002 from http://www.tdh.state.tx.us/hivstd/stats/pdf/qr20024.pdf .

United States Census (2000) [Online]. Retrieved on September 14, 2002 from http://www.census.gov.

Willard, C. L., Liljestrand, P., Goldschmidt, R. H., & Grumbach, K. (1999). Is experience with human immunodeficiency virus disease related to clinical practice? A survey of rural primary care physicians. *Archives of Family Medicine, 8*, 502-508.

doi:10.1300/J187v05n02_07

An Exploratory Study of HIV Prevention with Mexican/Latino Migrant Day Laborers

Kurt C. Organista, PhD
Nicholas J. Alvarado, MPH
Amity Balblutin-Burnham, MPH, MBA
Paula Worby, MPH
Sergio R. Martinez, BS

SUMMARY. The purpose of this exploratory study was to develop, implement, and evaluate a pilot HIV prevention intervention with one of the most mobile of U.S.-Mexico transborder populations: Mexican/Latino migrant day laborers (MDLs). Intervention development was informed

Kurt C. Organista, PhD, is Associate Professor at the School of Social Welfare, University of California, Berkeley, CA.

Nicholas J. Alvarado, MPH, is PAETC Minority Programs Manager, Department of Family and Community Medicine, University of California, San Francisco, CA.

Amity Balblutin-Burnham, MPH, MBA, is HIV Testing and Street Outreach Coordinator, City of Berkeley HIV/AIDS Program, Department of Health and Human Services, Berkeley, CA.

Paula Worby, MPH, is doctoral candidate, School of Public Health, University of California, Berkeley, CA.

Sergio R. Martinez, BS, is Community Health Outreach Worker, City of Berkeley HIV/AIDS Program, Department of Health and Human Services, Oakland, CA.

Address correspondence to: Kurt C. Organista, PhD, School of Social Welfare, 120 Haviland Hall, University of California, Berkeley, CA 94720-7400 (E-mail: DRKCO@ Berkeley.edu).

Partial funding for this project was provided by the Center for Latino Policy Research at the University of California, Berkeley.

[Haworth co-indexing entry note]: "An Exploratory Study of HIV Prevention with Mexican/Latino Migrant Day Laborers." Organista, Kurt C. et al. Co-published simultaneously in *Journal of HIV/AIDS & Social Services* (The Haworth Press, Inc.) Vol. 5, No. 2, 2006, pp. 89-114; and: *Outreach and Care Approaches to HIV/AIDS Along the US-Mexico Border* (ed: Herman Curiel, and Helen Land) The Haworth Press, Inc., 2006, pp. 89-114. Single or multiple copies of this article are available for a fee from The Haworth Document Delivery Service [1-800-HAWORTH, 9:00 a.m. - 5:00 p.m. (EST). E-mail address: docdelivery@haworthpress. com].

Available online at http://jhaso.haworthpress.com
© 2006 by The Haworth Press, Inc. All rights reserved.
doi:10.1300/J187v05n02_08

by preliminary research that included an HIV risk survey of over a hundred MDLs, and a focus group to explore the topic of HIV in the lives of MDLs. Both quantitative and qualitative methods were used to evaluate the intervention, and to identify some of the contextual characteristics of HIV risk factors in the MDL experience. For example, the most frequent theme revealed by qualitative analysis was the stressful and vulnerable state of *desesperación* [desperation], resulting from earning too little money, that participants linked to deviating from their migration goals and succumbing to alcohol and drug use, and risky sex. While empirical results are limited by the small sample of convenience ($N = 23$), lack of a control group, and loss of about half of the sample by one month follow-up evaluation, findings were encouragingly consistent with intervention goals: Post-intervention data revealed what appear to be substantial gains in carrying condoms (e.g., from 43% to 83%) as well as in knowledge of proper condom use. Further, frequency of sex with risky sex partners decreased in general, while condom use was reported for *all* sexual encounters assessed during post-evaluation. The theoretical framework used to guide the intervention, a hybrid of the Health Belief Model and Friere's model of participatory education, included visual triggers composed of customized Mexican lottery game cards to elicit discussion of HIV risk and prevention in the MDL experience. doi:10.1300/J187v05n02_08

[Article copies available for a fee from The Haworth Document Delivery Service: 1-800-HAWORTH. E-mail address: <docdelivery@haworthpress.com> Website: <http://www.HaworthPress.com> © 2006 by The Haworth Press, Inc. All rights reserved.]

KEYWORDS. HIV/AIDS, Mexicans, Latinos, Migrants, U.S.-Mexico border

This paper describes the development, implementation, and evaluation of a culturally responsive pilot study to prevent HIV risk in one of the most mobile trans-border populations to traverse the U.S.-Mexico border: Mexican/Latino migrant day laborers (MDLs).

HIV/AIDS RISK
IN MEXICAN/LATINO MIGRANT LABORERS

Reviews of the literature on HIV risk and Mexican/Latino migrant laborers describe a heterogeneous population at risk for various psychosocial and health problems due to a variety of factors related to both the nature of migratory labor in America, as well as to the demographic and cultural background characteristics of migrants themselves (Organista & Balls Organista, 1997; Organista, Carrillo, & Ayala, 2004). Worldwide migratory labor systems play significant roles in the geographical spread of HIV due to the predominance of young male laborers living and working far from home for extended periods of time, and consequent family breakdown, with increased number of sexual partners, including sex with female commercial sex workers and sex between men, consequently risking wives and other sex partners of migrant men.

Migration-Related HIV/AIDS Risk Factors

Documented HIV risk factors and co-factors for Mexican migrant laborers include high number of sex partners, significant rates of STDs, needle sharing following injections of illegal drugs as well as "therapeutic" self-injections of vitamins and antibiotics (Organista & Balls Organista, 1997), significant rates of alcohol and substance dependency, depression, and anxiety (Alderete, Vega, Kolody, & Aguilar-Gaxiola, 2000). Such risk factors are exacerbated by migratory labor that is generally difficult, inconsistent and low paying, exploitative, and frequently dangerous, lonely, and disruptive of normal social, romantic, and sexual relations.

Migrant background characteristics that further exacerbate HIV risk include low formal education and literacy rates, limited English proficiency, significant rates of undocumented status, low access to health and social services in the U.S., and traditional gender roles. While literature on migrant farmworkers and HIV risk is slowly beginning to accrue (e.g., Mishra, Conner, & Magana, 1996; Organista, 2004), far less is known about urban-based migrant laborers such as MDLs and those working in the vast service sector.

Migrant Day Laborers

According to Valenzuela (2003), day labor is defined as informal or non-standard work performed mostly by foreign-born Latino migrant men who congregate in "open air" markets, such as street corners or the parking lots of hardware stores, to solicit temporary daily work. Despite the rapid and continuing growth of MDLs in large and mid-sized urban centers of America, neither the U.S. Department of Labor nor the Bureau of the Census include day labor in their official classifications of work.

In his 1999 survey of 481 male MDLs from 87 different sites in Southern California, Valenzuela (2000) found the following background characteristics: predominantly Mexican (77%) and secondarily Central American (20%), 84% undocumented, less than five years in the U.S., average of 34 years of age, 50% married or living with partner, and an average of 7 years of education. With regard to work, the men averaged 4-5 days per week, 10% held regular jobs in addition to day labor; 43% had done day labor for less than a year; 31% for 2-5 years, and 20% between 6-10 years. When asked why they performed day labor, participants answered: because they lacked papers (40.3%), could not speak English (21%), and because regular jobs were scarce and paid too little money (18.2%). The men averaged about $7 an hour, with annual earnings of $8,489, and were generally paid in cash.

Valenzuela (2003) notes unregulated work with undocumented MDLs can result in frequent employer abuse. For example, over 50% of the men in his survey report being cheated out of wages, and there are also above average rates of injury and death resulting from performance of dangerous construction work without proper preparation, equipment, and supervision (Valenzuela, 2000). Significant stress, health and mental health problems are likely in such a socially, culturally, and legally marginalized population, living in urban-based poverty.

PRELIMINARY BACKGROUND RESEARCH

Assessment of HIV Risk in Local MDLs

Survey. Assessing HIV risk in 102 local MDLs began with the development of the Latino Migrant Laborer Questionnaire (LMLQ) designed to assess: (1) HIV risk related to sexual and substance use; (2) related psychosocial issues and problems affecting MDLs (e.g., problems encountered during the past six months); and (3) condom-related behaviors, knowledge, beliefs, and norms. While a full report of survey findings is available elsewhere (Organista & Kubo, 2005), an overview of key findings, with emphasis on their implications for the pilot prevention intervention, is listed in Table 1. As can be seen, survey participants resembled Valenzuela's (2000) MDL sample in background characteristics, and evidenced many of the same sex and substance use related HIV risk factors documented in the literature for Mexican migrant laborers in general (e.g., low and inconsistent condom use with a variety of sex partners; high rates of alcohol consumption, etc.).

TABLE 1. Overview of Findings from Preliminary HIV Risk Survey with MDLs (N = 102) with Implications for Development of HIV Prevention Intervention Group

Key survey findings	Implications for HIV prevention
1. Participants were primarily Spanish speaking Mexicans (two-thirds) and Central Americans; low in SES and acculturation to the U.S.; wages averaged between $100 and $400 a week, 40% of which was sent back home.	Conduct intervention in Spanish and provide financial incentives and meals for each session and evaluation.
2. Major psychosocial stressors reported during the past 6 months: a) Significant unemployment and underemployment b) Racism, social isolation, sadness, and loneliness c) Health problems without health care	Address HIV risk within the context of the often stressful MDL experience.
3. High rates of alcohol use and binge drinking that co-occur with sexual activities, and between 10% and 20% reported the additional use of marijuana, cocaine, and crack cocaine.	Address links between alcohol, substance use, sexual activity and HIV risk.
4. While only 7% of men reported illegal injection drug use, these men reported frequently sharing needles and rarely cleaning needles with bleach.	Address the role of needle sharing in HIV transmission.
5. Condom use was low and inconsistent, men generally did not carry condoms, and knowledge of proper condom use was poor. Men did report confidence in being able to insist on condom use in challenging sexual situations (e.g., when a sex partner does not want to use condoms), and they also reported frequent pro-condom attitudes and behaviors within their MDL circles.	Provide "hands-on" condom demonstrations with phallic replicas; urge men to carry condoms by building upon their reported pro-condom attitudes and confidence in using condoms.
6. Just over half of participants reported being sexually active during the past two months; and sexual activity with female partners was almost evenly divided between regular sex partners, including spouses, on the one hand, and one time only sex partners, including prostitutes, on the other.	Address safer sex strategies in response to sexual needs and with different types of sex partners in both the U.S. and country of origin.
7. No sex between men, or with transvestites/ transgendered persons, was reported, perhaps due to survey method of data collection.	Address ways in which sex between men occur among MDLs (e.g., being propositioned, homosexuality, etc.)
8. Efforts by MDLs to reduce HIV risk included: Higher condom use with one time only partners, including prostitutes and multiple sex partners; greater condom use during vaginal sex versus oral sex; and less oral sex with one time only partners, including prostitutes, and multiple sex partners.	Build upon such safer sex practices.
9. While HIV infection was not assessed, one third of the men reported a history of STDs such as syphilis and gonorrhea.	Provide education about HIV within the broader context of STDs.

Focus group. Following the survey, a semi-structured focus group was conducted with 13 MDLs to supplement survey findings with qualitative information on HIV risk within the local MDL experience. The community health clinic is located three short blocks from where the MDLs congregate to seek day labor, and is well-known for providing basic outpatient health care to local residents, especially poor residents without health insurance or income.

On the day of the focus group, the men were met on the corner and escorted to the clinic while they joked nervously about being turned over to *la migra* [slang for the INS]. Facilitators welcomed the men and explained the purpose of the group. The focus group began by asking participants to share names, origin, and reason for coming to the U.S., including good and bad experiences. Next, MDLs were asked to share: (1) what they know about HIV/AIDS, including risky situations observed and experienced; (2) whether they see links between HIV risk and their experiences as MDLs; and (3) what they've done or could do to lower HIV risk.

All focus group participants shared the common migration theme of coming the U.S. to earn money and help their families, while simultaneously encountering considerable stress and vulnerability to *caerse en los vicios* [falling into the vices] such as excessive drinking, occasional drug use, and unprotected sex. While the men were forthcoming about sex with female sex workers and occasional *amantes* [lovers] in the U.S., they did not discuss sex between men until asked. One man mentioned being propositioned by a man who hired him to do yard work, and added that he would have traded sex for the extra $50 offered had he been financially desperate.

Implications for intervention. Survey implications for intervention ranged from providing training on correct condom use to addressing links between the MDL experience, stress, alcohol and substance use, and unprotected sex with a variety of female partners. Focus group implications for intervention were similar but also included the need for facilitators to push the topic of sex between men and the different ways it happens in the MDL experience. The focus group also confirmed sufficient enthusiasm on the part of MDLs to participate in a longer and more structured HIV prevention group, provided that culturally competent and trustful relationships, financial incentives, and a flexible schedule were in place. More pragmatic lessons learned included recruiting men who earn most of their income from day labor (one focus group participant reported using day labor to supplement full-time work), and asking participants to refrain from alcohol and/or substance use prior to intervention (one man smelled of alcohol).

Theoretical framework. Based on the lessons learned above, as well as pertinent literature, it was decided to employ a theoretical framework composed of a hybrid of the Health Beliefs Model, pervasive in the field of HIV prevention, and the increasingly popular participatory education model of Brazilian educator Paolo Friere. The HBM model predicts that people will protect their health provided that they are aware of a particular health risk (e.g., HIV), possess the skills to prevent the health risk (e.g., condom use), and feel confident that implementing such skills will be effective (Glanz, Marcus Lewis, & Rimer, 1997). However, Friere (1970) cautions, especially when working with oppressed groups, that well-meaning professionals may inadvertently recapitulate dynamics of oppression if, in their roles as experts, they speak down to and impose their knowledge and recommendations upon members of at-risk groups. Thus, he recommends that while professionals should provide basic education and technical assistance, especially when requested by community members, they should concentrate their efforts on facilitating a process of active problem identification, definition, and problem-solving on the part of the group's members whom they are trying to help. Wallerstein (1992) argues further that health education with limited-English skills should rely less on written materials, employ culturally appropriate approaches, and should engage participants in the learning process following a Freirian problem-posing model. Further, Wallerstein notes that such an approach should use visual or story triggers that prompt open-ended discussion.

An example of such a story trigger, used in the current study to prompt open-ended discussion about MDLs and HIV risk, is the vignette described as follows. Examples of visual triggers, used to elicit discussion of more specific MDL-related HIV risk factors, are the poster-sized Mexican lottery game cards developed specifically for the intervention group. *Loteria* is a traditional Mexican card game like bingo except that in addition to numbers, each playing card contains 16 tarot card-like images that are very familiar to Mexicans. For example, the *El Borracho* [the drunk] card depicts a hunched-over intoxicated Mexican man, the *La Muerte* [death] card depicts the Grim Reaper, and *La Escalera* [the ladder] depicts a ladder that can be viewed as symbolizing progress (see Figure 1). The above images were reproduced from actual Mexican game cards while others were created by the research team to depict HIV/AIDS issues raised in the focus group such as *La Prostituta* [the prostitute], *La Amante* [the lover], and *Sexo entre Hombres* [sex be-

FIGURE 1. Loteria for HIV Prevention

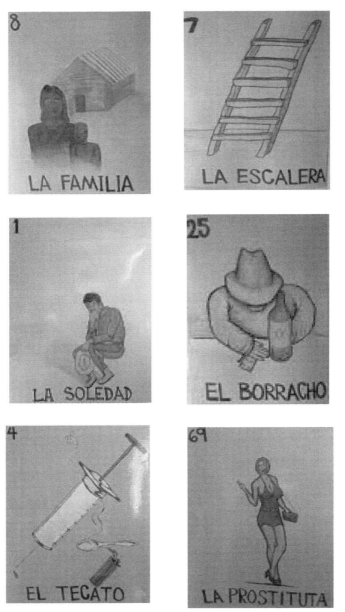

Note: Artwork by Ari Haytin, Street outreach worker, City of Berkeley HIV/AIDS Program. Printed with permission.

tween men]. These visual triggers, hung on the walls of the group intervention room, were effective in eliciting spontaneous comments from men about the *vicios* [vices] encountered, and were used to direct men's attention to risk factors under discussion.

The idea of using culturally familiar forms of Mexican entertainment to facilitate HIV prevention also came from a pair of auspicious prevention interventions with Mexican farm workers, successful in increasing condom use with female sex workers by utilizing Mexican-style *Fotonovelas* [dramatic and humorous comic book-like novellas that use actual photos and bubble dialogue] and *Radionovelas* [radio broadcasted mini soap operas] to depict three scenarios in which a male farm worker respectively: (1) uses a condom with a prostitute; (2) abstains from sex with the prostitute; (3) infects wife and child with HIV as a result of unprotected sex with the prostitute (Mishra & Connor, 1996; Sanudo, 1999). Such popular forms of Mexican entertainment are simultaneously funny and melodramatic on the one hand, yet dead serious on the other. Thus, such Mexican media can provide a culturally familiar way of addressing the serious business of HIV/AIDS.

Development of the Pilot HIV Prevention Intervention

A three-session HIV prevention group, designed to meet at convenient times within the span of a week, was developed given the transient nature of the study population. Table 2 provides an overview of the intervention group's objectives and methods, as well as outcomes observed by group facilitators.

For example, *objectives* for Session 1 included orientation regarding the purpose of the group, personal introductions and, consistent with the HBM, raising awareness of HIV risk in MDLs. *Methods* for Session 1 included giving each participant the opportunity to tell his migration story; and observed *outcomes* included group cohesion and identification of MDL-related stressors and HIV risks. *Objectives* for Session 2 included providing an opportunity to answer any question about HIV/AIDS, and increasing skills to reduce HIV risk (e.g., correct condom use, ways to avoid or respond to risky sexual situations). *Methods* for Session 2 included condom use demonstration and hands-on practice with phallic replicas; and *outcomes* included correcting misconceptions about HIV transmission, and raising confidence in condom use by correcting improper use (e.g., putting condom on phallic replicas correctly). Session 2 *objectives* also included identifying personal HIV risks actually experienced by participants, facilitated by asking partici-

TABLE 2. Overview of HIV Prevention Intervention Group for Latino Migrant Day laborers

	Objectives	Methods	Outcomes
Session 1	–To explain rationale and purpose of study –To engage participants in group process –Assess and increase awareness regarding risk for HIV/AIDS among MDLs –To hear the personal stories of each participant –To build a sense of community throughout	–Use *Personalismo* to build rapport & trust and share goal of reducing HIV risk in MDLs –Provide cash incentives, meals, comfortable group setting; discuss ground rules for a productive group –Provide opportunity for each participant to share his MDL story (migration goals and obstacles) –Use customized Mexican lottery cards as visual triggers to elicit discussion of HIV risk related to MDL experience	–Participants gratified to hear facilitators express concern for MDLs –Each participant shared migration story and discovered much in common with others --Risks for HIV were identified as well as stressors related to MDL experience
Session 2	–To increase knowledge about HIV/AIDS & STDs –To increase HIV prevention skills (e.g., correct condom use) –To identify and discuss HIV risk scenarios for each participant	–Provide basic HIV/AIDS/STD education –Use vignette as story trigger to elicit discussion of HIV risk in MDLs' experience –Condom demonstration and hands-on practice with phallic replicas	–Men very interested in HIV education, misconceptions versus inaccurate information –Men learned correct condom use after demonstrating many mistakes –Men fairly forthcoming with respect to HIV risks personally encountered and observed
Session 3	–To review salient MDL HIV risk scenarios from previous session –To have participants generate different ways of managing HIV risk –To solicit feedback and suggestions regarding the group –To provide closure to group experience	–Pose various HIV risk related problems and scenarios, based on information from previous sessions –Have each participant brainstorm various strategies to reduce HIV risk –Solicit group feedback regarding each participant's risk reduction ideas –Continue using lottery cards as visual triggers to elicit discussion about specific HIV risk factors –Ask each participant to name one or two helpful things from the group, and to share any other thoughts, feelings, recommendations, etc.	–Men tended to repeat what they learned in previous session rather than personalizing their own risks –Men planned to reduce risk by "using condoms" but needed to be challenged by posing challenging situations –Group provided good feedback regarding the feasibility of each participant's HIV risk reduction ideas (e.g., recent arrivals relying on abstinence were challenged by seasoned MDLs) –Men were impressed with education component of group, chance to speak to each other –Men expressed much gratitude for group experience

	Objectives	Methods	Outcomes
Follow-up	−Assess changes in HIV-related risk behavior since participating in group	−Administer four week post-intervention evaluation questionnaire to group participants	−12 of 23 men returned for or were located for post-intervention assessment

pants their reactions to the following story trigger (developed from a composite of various HIV-positive MDLs treated by clinic staff):

> *Andres was a jornalero of 23 years who arrived in the U.S. a year-and-a-half ago, with all good intentions. He came to El Norte to financially help out his family back in Mexico, lived in San Francisco with five other MDLs who engaged in high-risk behaviors for HIV. They were injecting drugs, one was dealing drugs, and one began to hustle sex on Polk Street when he needed extra cash. The men slept together due to a shortage of beds and space. Because Andres was not finding enough work and pay, he fell into his roommate's vices. He was vulnerable, became desperate, and ultimately became infected with HIV.*

For one recently arrived participant, the above story triggered the response that he didn't need to carry condoms because he had no intention of having sex while in the U.S. Immediately another MDL with years in the U.S. said that he should still carry condoms "just in case" because he felt the same when he first came to the U.S., only to eventually succumb to sexual temptations.

Consistent with Friere, *Objectives* for Session 3 centered on reducing HIV risk by posing various risk-related problems to the group, as well as to specific individuals, based on all that was learned and discussed in previous sessions. For example, "Suppose you're broke, and feeling desperate, and a man hires you to clean his yard but later offers you $50 for a sexual favor. What could you do in this situation to reduce risk for HIV?" Individual participants were given the opportunity to problem-solve such risk scenarios, by brainstorming various strategies, followed by asking the other group participants what they thought about such strategies.

The Current Study

The purpose of the current exploratory study was to implement and evaluate the above HIV prevention pilot group for MDLs. In terms of outcome variables, the group was primarily intended to: (1) decrease risky sex with a variety of sex partners (i.e., decrease frequency of sex with risky partners as well as increase condom use when having sex); and (2) increase correct condom use knowledge and skills. While not a direct focus of the intervention, the research team wondered if the intervention would have any effect on alcohol and substance use (e.g., if discussions linking HIV risk to excessive drinking would decrease such alcohol use). Both quantitative and qualitative methods were also employed to capture specific HIV risk factors and their various contexts in the MDL experience. The following exploratory research questions were addressed in this study: (1) What are some of the contextual characteristics of HIV risk in the MDL experience? (2) Will the HIV prevention group indirectly decrease alcohol and substance use? (3) Will the HIV prevention group improve condom use knowledge and skills? and (4) Will the HIV prevention group decrease the frequency of risky sex (e.g., with sex workers, one time only partners), as well as increase the frequency of condom use when having sex?

METHODS

Participants

Participants were 23 MDLs who participated in two HIV prevention groups (11 in the first group and 12 in the second) with background characteristics very similar to those reported in the above survey: 70% Mexican origin, 26% Central American, 4% other, with a very low level of acculturation to U.S. (e.g., predominantly monolingual Spanish speaking). Just under half were married (48%), 39% single, and 3% divorced. The men averaged four years in the U.S., and 34 years of age (SD = 9.5). With regards to income, 78% reported earning between $100 and $400 a week, while the remaining indicated less than $100 a week. Participants reported sending 49% of their income back home to family in Mexico or Central America.

Procedures

Recruitment. For each of the two intervention groups, a small convenience sample of MDLs was recruited from the street corner where they seek day labor. Men were approached by outreach workers who screened for the following inclusion criteria: 18 years or older, earning majority of income from day labor, able to commit to the three scheduled group sessions and one month follow-up assessment, agreement to refrain from alcohol and/or substance use prior to intervention group sessions. Prospective participants were provided with attractive reminder cards listing intervention dates, times, locations, and increasing cash incentives for each of the three sessions ($20, $25, $30), and for the one month post-evaluation ($30). Reminder cards included a contact person's name and phone number. On the day of the first group session, recruits were met on the corner and escorted to the clinic.

A short version of the LMLQ was used for the pre- and four week post-intervention follow-up evaluations. Pre-assessment evaluation was conducted in the field during recruitment (about a week prior to Session 1). The decision to conduct the follow-up evaluation four weeks after the intervention was made in the hope of not losing too many of these mobile participants, while still allowing a window of time to transpire in which to assess possible behavioral change.

Group participation. For both groups combined, 23 men began the intervention, 17 completed it, and 12 either returned for the four-week post-intervention evaluation, or were located by research team members (e.g., by visiting the corner where the MDLs seek work, leaving messages at the phone number left by some participants, and by asking post-evaluation completers to remind the others to return).

Measures

Selected LMLQ items and scales are described below. Given the small sample size, the psychometric properties of scales are reported for the above MDL survey where appropriate.

Acculturation. Level of acculturation to the U.S. was assessed by four language-related items that compose the language factor of the Short Acculturation Scale ([SAS], Marín, Sabogal, Marín, Otero-Sabogal, & Pérez-Stable, 1987). For example, participants are asked, "What language do you read and speak? . . . speak with friends?," etc. These items are arranged on five-point scales ranging from "Only Spanish" [1] to "Only English" [5], with "Both equally" [3] as a mid-point. This factor had a mean of 1.3 (*SD* = .56) indicating very low acculturation to the U.S. In the above MDL survey, this scale had essentially the same mean score (1.5), as well as a *coefficient alpha* of .73, indicating fair internal consistency reliability. It should be noted that while this four-item language factor is only one of several dimensions of acculturation assessed by the SAS, it does account for most of the scale's variance and is thus commonly used in place of the full scale (i.e., the other dimensions add little to the variance in SAS scores).

Alcohol and substance use. Alcohol use during the past month was assessed by an item asking about the frequency with which alcoholic beverages were consumed: never, 1-3 times/month, 1-2 times/week, 3-4 times a week, everyday, and more than once a day. A follow-up item asked about the number of alcoholic beverages consumed on a typical day of drinking. Five items were used to assess the frequency with which participants used the following illegal drugs during the past month: marijuana, cocaine, crack cocaine, amphetamines, and heroin. The same six-point scale used to assess alcohol intake was used. These five illegal drugs were assessed because they were the only ones used from a longer list used in the MDL survey.

Condom-related knowledge, efficacy and social norms. Knowledge of proper condom use was assessed by three items ("Do you think Vaseline is a good lubricant for condoms?" "Is it necessary to unroll a condom before putting it on the penis?" and "Is it necessary to grab the condom while withdrawing the penis after ejaculating?"), previously used with samples of Mexican migrant laborers (Organista et al., 1997). An eight-item condom-related social norm scale assessed the frequency with which respondents, together with their friends and family members, condone condom use in a variety of ways. For example, respondents were asked how frequently they and their friends and family members: recommend, criticize, give, and ask for condoms. Items are scored on four-point scales ranging from 1 (Very frequently) to 4 (Never), and the scale had very good internal consistency reliability (*coefficient alpha* = .87) in the MDL survey.

The condom efficacy scale consisted of 17 items that assessed how confident respondents feel about negotiating condom use with partners in a variety of challenging sexual situations. For example, interviewees were asked how capable they would be of insisting on condom use if a prospective sex partner were to: get angry, not want to use a condom, threaten to leave, etc. Other items assessed condom use capability with a sex partner with whom the respondent was in love, who was using another form of birth control, who wanted to have a baby, etc. These items were scored on five-point scales ranging from 1 (Definitely no) to 5 (Definitely yes) with 3 (Maybe) as a mid-point. In the MDL survey, this scale also had good internal consistency as indicated by a coefficient alpha of .85.

Sexual activities and partners. This was the first of three matrices constructed to assess various types of sexual partners and activities during the past month. Participants were asked: "During the past month, with how many *women* have you had sex?" ". . . with how many *men* have you had sex?" and ". . . with how many *transsexuals or transvestites* have you had sex (men who dress like women or who have changed their sex)?" If participants answer yes to any of the above items, they are asked these follow-up questions: "Of these persons, with how many did you have sex only one time?" "How many of these were regular partners, lovers, girlfriend/boyfriend?" "How many were prostitutes?" and (where applicable) "Was one of these persons your spouse?"

Sex between men and women. Next, participants were asked about the following sexual behaviors in heterosexual relations: "During the past month, have you had vaginal sex (the penis in the vagina)?" ". . . have you had anal sex (the penis in the anus)?" ". . . have you had oral sex (the penis in the mouth)?" and ". . . have you had oral sex (the mouth/tongue on the vagina)?" If participants answer yes to any, they are asked these follow-up questions: "With or without condoms?" (with or without dental dam in the case of mouth to vagina oral sex), "Of these persons, with how many did you have sex only one time?" "How many of these were regular partners, lovers, girlfriends/boyfriends?" "How many were prostitutes?" "Was one of these persons your spouse?" and "With how many did you exchange sex for money, drugs, a place to sleep, or something else?"

Sex between men. Finally, participants were asked about the following sexual behaviors in homosexual relations between men: "During the past month, have you had insertive oral sex (your penis in his mouth)?" ". . . have you had receptive oral sex (his penis in your mouth)?" ". . . have you had insertive anal sex (your penis in his anus)?" ". . . have you had receptive anal sex (his penis in your anus)?" If the answer to any of the above items is yes, participants are asked these follow-up questions: "With or without condoms?" "With how many men?" "Of these men, with how many did you have sex only one time?" "How many of these were regular partners, lovers, or boyfriends?" "How many were prostitutes?" and ". . . with how many did you exchange sex for money, drugs, a place to sleep, or something else?"

Data Analysis

Given the small sample of convenience, basic descriptive statistics such as percentages and mean scores are used to compare pre- and post-intervention quantitative data. With regard to qualitative data, tape recordings from the second intervention group were transcribed and analyzed by a team member to document how session interactions transpired and to elucidate themes to guide further intervention development. Approximately four and a half hours of audiotape were transcribed resulting in about 80 pages of narrative. One of the group facilitators had taken notes during the intervention and reviewed the transcript to match persons to quotes in order to better track the trains of thought expressed by different participants.

Qualitative analysis used codes developed from repeated and close readings of the transcripts instead of using predetermined or template codes (Addison, 1999; Crabtree & Miller, 1999). These codes were later refined throughout the process to capture the significant themes emerging from the group discussion. The next step was to piece together participant stories, mostly from their introductory statements, to give each participant a voice and identity. An introductory paragraph about each participant was then followed by all the quotes that had been identified for that person. This method allowed for a "vertical" analysis of the themes emerging from each speaker alongside information about the speaker's background. The quotes were then grouped by codes. Quotes that could and could not be attributed to any speaker were regrouped under themes, allowing for a "horizontal" analysis and further refining of codes.

There was no attempt to analyze qualitative data as those of the individuals per se within the group, given that the group itself would be considered the unit of analysis and opinions and themes emerging in the group are not independent from one another. Nevertheless, the emerging themes, ideas, and the language used by participants add texture and *speak with* quantitative results, as described below. Given the limited length of transcripts, data analysis was feasible through multiple readings and coding of the text without the aid of software.

RESULTS

Results of qualitative and quantitative data analysis are integrated below in order to describe some of the contextual characteristics of HIV risk in the MDL experience, and to convey how both methods of data analysis mutually inform or *speak to* each other.

Contextual Characteristics of HIV Risk in the MDL Experience

Results of qualitative data analysis show that participants are concerned, first and foremost, about obtaining work and wages in order to secure their immediate livelihood and to support their very identity as laborers who endure the hardship of leaving their families behind in order to provide for them. The sacrifice of leaving families is great and can either be what keeps them going or, during hard times, brings them to despair:

> *So basically we have to leave our whole family, we leave a wife, we leave our children–in my case I have two daughters for whom I have to look out for, at least so they can get some kind of job training, so that in the future they will have a way to get ahead.*

> *. . . Like now when you really want to go see your family and you get desperate about it.*

With regard to how stress, related to the MDL experience, is linked to risk, *Desesperación* [despair] came up repeatedly as a favored term to describe the painful and vulnerable state of mind that results from not satisfying one's main goal as a migrant laborer. While despair is viewed as an effect of too little money, it is also viewed as strong enough to push the men over the edge into risky behaviors. The men described a causal chain or slippery slope from sadness, loneliness and desperation to excessive drinking and drug use, and no longer caring about important things. This idea was the single most frequent theme:

> *But sometimes it is difficult to get work and then the desperation, the loneliness that one finds in this country! You know what I mean? The loneliness, you shut yourself in a room with four walls . . . you come to this country and sometimes you have no friends, nobody to talk with. You are all alone and at times, even if you come and have relatives here, a cousin or someone, they turn their back on you. They don't help you. You can get to the point where you don't have anything, not even to eat . . . you feel so desperate, so upset. You walk along and don't know what to do you are so desperate.*

> *It's like others are saying: desperation because I don't get much work. The desperation and also drinking. Drinking and drugs and that's how I was here. . . . I have just been here a year but I get so desperate and I have to get out. I'm in the house watching TV and I am desperate to go or do something so I go out and walk in Berkeley.*

The idea of a slippery slope was reinforced by imagery of how one either "fell" into vices or problems or stayed on the straight and narrow either with the help of friends and relatives in the U.S. or by being in frequent contact with one's family back home:

> *The reason I came to the U.S. was to look for a better life, supposedly, but once you're here, there are all kinds of problems like loneliness, depression, separation from your family. One can fall into depression and when you're depressed, then you resort to alcoholism and drugs. And then you get more problems. You can forget the reason you came here in the first place.*

> *So here I am suffering because I can't get work and now it's been about 10 days since I've gotten work and at times I get really desperate–like the others are saying–that I don't find work but thank God that my pal rents me a room because there are so many guys who don't have anyone and they end up sleeping in the street and fall into vices. They start drinking–precisely because they have no work–and they get into drugs.*

Alcohol and Substance Use

Despite the many references above to alcohol and substance use as outcomes of desesperación, the intervention appeared to have no impact on this important problem area. For example, pre- and post-intervention alcohol rates hardly vary at different levels of use during the past month: None (30% & 33%, respectively), between 1-3 drinks/month and 1-2 drinks/week (52% & 50%, respectively), and between 3-4 drinks/week and more than one drink a day (18% & 16%, respectively). The same pre- and post-assessment pattern was found for Marijuana at different levels of use: None (70% & 75%, respectively); 1-3 times/month (22% & 17%, respectively), 1-2 times/week (0% & 8%), and 3-4 times/week (9% & 0%). Use of heroin, amphetamine, cocaine, and crack was negligible at both pre- and post-assessment.

Condom Knowledge and Behaviors

As can be seen in Table 3, frequency of carrying condoms, and gains in knowledge of proper condom use, were encouraging. For example, when asked about frequency of carrying condoms, only 43% of men said "Always" at pre-intervention as compared to twice that percentage

TABLE 3. Condom Knowledge and Behaviors in Latino Migrant Day Laborers

Items	Pre (N = 23) Mean	Post (N = 12) Mean
Frequency of Carrying Condoms		
Always	43%	83%
Sometimes	22%	17%
Almost never	9%	0%
Never	26%	0%
Knowledge of Correct Condom Use		
Vaseline good lubricant for condoms?		
Correct	30%	58%
Incorrect/Unknown	43%	33%
Unroll condom before putting on penis?		
Correct	74%	83%
Incorrect/Unknown	17%	8%
Grab condom while withdrawing after coming?		
Correct	57%	92%
Incorrect/Unknown	22%	8%
Condom Social Norm[1] (M)	2.5	2.5
Condom Efficacy[2] (M)	1.7	1.2

Note: 1: 1 = Very frequently & 4 = Never; 2: 1 = Definitely yes; 3 = Sometimes; 5 = Definitely no

at post-assessment. Similarly, a quarter of participants reported "Never" carrying condoms at pre-assessment as compared to 0% at post-assessment. Gains in knowledge of proper condom use also doubled from pre- to post-assessment on two of the condom knowledge items, while increasing by 9% on the third item. While the lack of change on condom-related norms is not surprising, given the social context of this variable, there appeared to be slight improvement on condom self-efficacy: from a mean of 1.7 ("Yes") to 1.2 ("Definitely yes") when asked about confidence in insisting on condom use in challenging sexual situations.

Sexual Partners and Behaviors

As can be seen in Table 4, the general pattern of results for HIV risk related to sexual partners and behaviors reveals two encouraging trends.

TABLE 4. Vaginal Sex and Condom Use During the Past Month

	Pre-With Condoms	Pre-Without Condoms	Post-With Condoms	Post-Without Condoms
	N (23)	N (23)	N (12)	N (12)
Total number of women				
1	26%	39%	25%	0%
2	0%	0%	0%	0%
3 or more	4%	4%	8%	0%
One time only partners?				
1	22%	17%	8%	0%
2	0%	4%	0%	0%
3 or more	0%	0%	0%	0%
Regular partners?				
1	13%	17%	25%	0%
2 or more	0%	4%	0%	0%
Prostitutes?				
1	9%	17%	0%	0%
2	0%	4%	0%	0%
3 or more	0%	0%	0%	0%
Ever exchange sex for something?	4%	4%	8%	0%
Was one of the above your spouse?	0%	9%	0%	0%

The first trend is that none of the participants reported sex without condoms at post-intervention assessment as compared to 43% at pre-intervention assessment. For example, during the month prior to the intervention, 21% of men report no condom use during sex with: regular, one time only, and prostitute sex partners, as compared to 0% in the month after the intervention. The second trend is a decrease in the frequency of sex in general with all types of sex partners assessed. For example, 73% of men reported sex with between one and three or more sex partners at pre-intervention as compared to half as many at post-intervention. Further, no men reported sex with prostitutes in the month following the intervention as compared to just under a third at pre-intervention. Sex with one time only sex partners dropped from 43% at pre-intervention to 8% at post-intervention.

Qualitative results revealed that the main behavior that men felt was connected to STDs and HIV was sex with commercial sex workers. On the one hand men felt that sex with prostitutes was risky and cut into their savings and was therefore a waste of money for a brief moment of pleasure: "Better to masturbate, that way I won't go paying 20, 30 dollars." This was juxtaposed with sending this same money to your family: "So, not sending money home to your wife because you go with a woman . . ." On the other hand, either for men who are single or think that masturbation has its limits, spending the money is worth it as illustrated by this interchange:

> –*The problem is that here there are places that if you go, they'll charge you 160 [dollars], what you could earn in a week! It'd be better to go masturbate.*

> –*Well, what about going once every two or three months? Not every week!*

> –*I have seen lots [of guys], wow–something else! As soon as a week goes by and they have some cash–off they go!*

Men described being solicited by sex workers on the street and feeling like when the temptation is there, it takes will to resist because "The flesh is weak." One told the story of getting on the bus that very evening and having two sex workers "who spoke a little Spanish" tease and proposition him.

Qualitative findings shed light on the larger context of sex in the U.S. including links between sex workers, girlfriends, and wives back in their country of origin. For example, one man articulated an important reason why men like himself look to a prostitute for sex: worrying about cultural norms in the U.S. means that migrant men often aren't free to pursue girlfriends for fear of doing something wrong.

> *The problem is that at times you have to have relations with a prostitute because, what are you going to do? You can't flirt with someone because here before you know it they'll want to have the police after you. It is really different, you know?*

The comment above was immediately echoed by another participant. At least three men (all with wives and children back home) emphasized that fidelity to one's partner was possible and that masturbation could resolve their physical needs. Commitment to their partners and concern about becoming sick and infecting their partners were mentioned as reasons for avoiding sex workers, although, as the following quote shows, fear of disease might be seen as a more acceptable reason to abstain than the value of fidelity:

> *I don't think about [sexual risks] because, I don't know, perhaps because I love my wife or something like that but I don't think about it. . . . [And masturbation] is the safest form of sex because in addition to being faithful I'm scared about contracting one of these diseases. It's not that I'm so faithful to my wife, it's the risk of easily getting a disease.*

Interestingly, the same man commented that he is pressured or teased by other men for not "going with other women" but that he has held fast in his determination.

HIV/AIDS Knowledge and Concern

Qualitative findings suggest that sufficient trust developed in the group for participants to reveal their questions, and frequent misperceptions, about HIV and related topics. They asked about getting HIV from bathrooms, mosquitoes, and sharing utensils. One man related having "heard on TV" that masturbation can cause STDs, and another wanted to know if it was true that condoms came in different sizes. Another man cited an acquaintance who first gets oral sex performed on him "naturally" (with no condom) and then "does it" (vaginal sex) with a condom; and asked: what was the man's risk in this case? Such misconceptions about HIV/AIDS may be rooted in the low priority of this problem area relative to more immediate concerns. For example, one man spoke to the frequent threat of violence in the MDL experience:

> *There is also the risk that you get killed or risk getting robbed at least. Tonight I'll go right home to my room fast because robbers break in the rooms where we stay, they break in and before you know it, they'll kill you for just a little money and even if you don't have it, they'll beat you up. These are the risks we face . . . lots of risks!*

DISCUSSION

The purpose of this exploratory study was to develop, implement, and evaluate a small pilot HIV prevention intervention for Mexican/Latino MDLs, in preparation for larger and more rigorous intervention efforts. Preliminary background research included an HIV risk survey of 102 MDLs, and a focus group of 13 MDLs, to inform intervention development. As a result, perception of HIV risk and skills to reduce risk were enhanced (e.g., avoiding risky sex, condom use when engaging in sex). Discussions of HIV risk were facilitated by using story and visual triggers, while multiple strategies for reducing risk were generated by posing risk scenarios.

While results are not generalizable given the small sample of convenience, lack of a control group, and the loss of about half of the sample by follow-up evaluation, findings were encouragingly consistent with intervention goals, and warrant ongoing research. Mixed quantitative and qualitative evaluation methods were helpful in describing contextual characteristics of HIV risk factors in the MDL experience. For example, in response to the first study question, qualitative data analysis revealed how the central priority of earning enough money, for self and family, can result in a vulnerable state of desesperación given the frequent unemployment and underemployment that characterize migrant labor in the U.S. (Organista, 2004a). Participants linked such desperation to deviating from their migrant goals and succumbing to *vicios* such as excessive alcohol, occasional drug use, and risky sex. How the stress of desesperación forms a context for risk in general was the single most frequent theme that emerged from qualitative data analysis.

Regarding the second study question, the intervention appeared to have no impact on alcohol or substance use, most likely due to the lack of any specific focus on these HIV risk co-factors. Future efforts need to target this problem area more systematically (e.g., social integration efforts to decrease isolation and overreliance on drinking with fellow *jornaleros* as a way to relieve stress, meet affiliation needs, etc.).

Regarding the third study question, post-intervention data revealed what appear to be substantial gains in carrying condoms (e.g., from 43% to 83%) and knowledge of proper condom use. These findings suggest that intervention time devoted to demonstrating proper condom use, including "hands-on" practice with phallic replicas, was beneficial.

In view of the overriding objective of this study to decrease risky sexual behaviors, and to increase safer sex (i.e., condom use), it is noteworthy that pre- to post-intervention change suggested both of these desired trends: the frequency of risky sex (i.e., with one time only, multiple, and sex worker partners) decreased in general, while condom use was reported for *all* sexual encounters during the four weeks following intervention. Thus, results suggest that this type of intervention could decrease sexual risk-taking in MDLs.

Qualitative data analysis was helpful in contextualizing the (risky) sexual experiences of MDLs. For example, sex with sex workers was discussed frequently as a way to satisfy sexual needs, especially considering that MDLs are occasionally solicited by sex workers, and because many expressed difficulty in developing relationships with *amantes* or lovers in the U.S.

Married participants did discuss trying to be faithful to wives, if only to prevent the spread of HIV, through willpower, throwing themselves into work, masturbation, and considering the financial cost of sex workers. Such naturally occurring methods of risk reduction could be enhanced in future prevention efforts (e.g., cost-benefit analysis of using sex workers, discussion of risks posed to wives and other sex partners, etc.).

With regard to study limitations, 23 men began the three-session intervention and 17 (74%) were able to complete it within the span of a week. The fact that only half of the sample could be located for the four-week post-intervention evaluation is problematic and calls for improving follow-up evaluation by giving participants phone cards with which to call during the post-evaluation period, and providing them with postcards, addressed to the clinic, on which to indicate current whereabouts, to facilitate post-assessments (e.g., by phone, at new location).

Future MDL interventions will consider ways of more actively involving *jornaleros* in intervention efforts. For example, outstanding intervention completers (i.e., those especially involved and helpful to group process) could be asked to participate in a subsequent group as peer facilitators, and to assist with participant recruitment. Upon completing the intervention, facilitators were approached by at least one participant per group who asked if they could be of further assistance. For instance, in one of the groups, an out gay MDL spoke openly of his risk experiences, and assertively challenged other participants not to increase risk in Gay Latinos by ridiculing and rejecting them. By making statements such as "We are all men here with sexual needs and the need to protect ourselves," he eventually gained the respect of other participants who stopped their joking about homosexuals and even expressed respect for what he had to say.

CONCLUSION

Despite the stated limitations of this small pilot study, the promising pattern of results warrants larger and more rigorous tests of the intervention that blends theoretical elements of the health beliefs model and Friere's participatory education model, and includes the use of a popular form of Mexican entertainment as a culturally familiar visual trigger to facilitate problem conceptualization and risk reduction on the part of Mexican/Latino MDLs. With regard to practice, the engaging intervention model could also be incorporated into agency and community level efforts to prevent HIV in MDLs. Migrant day labor centers represent promising sites for not only organizing day labor but for also addressing the many psychosocial and health needs of MDLs, including HIV prevention. However, the development of such controversial centers (e.g., they are banned in Arizona) depends on advocacy at the local level to include MDLs in city and county health-related policies.

REFERENCES

Addison, R. B. (1999). A grounded hermeneutic editing approach. In W. L. Miller & B. F. Crabtree (Eds.), *Doing qualitative research* (pp. 145-161). Thousand Oaks, CA: Sage Publications.

Alderete, E., Vega, W. A., Kolody, B., & Aguilar-Gaxiola, S. (2000). Lifetime prevalence of risk factors for psychiatric disorders among Mexican migrant farmworkers in California. *American Journal of Public Health, 90*(4), 608-614.

Crabtree B. F., & Miller, W. L. (1999). Using codes and code manuals. In W. L. Miller & B. F. Crabtree (Eds.), *Doing qualitative research* (pp. 163-177). Thousand Oaks, CA: Sage Publications.

Friere, P. (1970). *Pedagogy of the oppressed* (Ramos, M. B., Trans.). New York: Continuum.

Glanz, K., Marcus Lewis, F., & Rimer, B. K. (Eds.) (1997). *Health behavior and health education: Theory research and practice* (2nd ed.). San Francisco: Jossey-Bass Inc.

Marín, G., Sabogal, F., Marín, B. V., Otero-Sabogal, R., & Pérez-Stable, E. J. (1987). Development of a short acculturation scale for Hispanics. *Hispanic Journal of Behavioral Science, 9*, 183-205.

Mishra, S. I., & Conner, R. F. (1996). Evaluation of an HIV prevention program among Latino farmworkers. In S. I. Mishra, R. F. Connor, & J. R. Magana (Eds.), *AIDS crossing borders: The spread of HIV among migrant Latinos* (pp. 157-181). Boulder, CO: Westview Press.

Mishra, S. I., Conner, R. F., & Magana, J. R. (1996). *AIDS crossing borders: The spread of HIV among migrant Latinos*. Boulder, CO: Westview Press.

Organista, K. C. (2004). HIV prevention models with Mexican farmworkers. In R. Mancoske (Ed.), *Practice models in HIV services* (pp. 127-160). New York: The Haworth Press, Inc.

Organista, K. C., & Balls Organista, P. (1997). Migrant laborers and AIDS in the United States: A review of the literature. *AIDS Education and Prevention, 9*, 83-93.

Organista, K. C., Balls Organista, P., Garcia de Alba G., J. E., Castillo Moran, M. A., & Ureta Carrillo, L. E. (1997). Survey of condom-related beliefs, behaviors, and perceived social norms in Mexican migrant laborers. *Journal of Community Health*, *22*(3), 185-198.

Organista, K. C., Carrillo, H., & Ayala, G. (2004). HIV prevention with Mexican migrants: Review, critique, and recommendations. *Journal of Acquired Immune Deficiency Syndrome*, *37* (Suppl. 4), S227-S239.

Organista, K. C., & Kubo, A. (2005). Pilot survey of HIV risk and contextual problems and issues in Mexican/Latino migrant day laborers. *Journal of Immigrant Health*, *7*(4), 269-281.

Sanudo, F. (1999). The effects of a culturally appropriate HIV intervention on Mexican farmworkers' knowledge, attitudes, and condom use behavior. Unpublished Master's Thesis. San Diego State University, Department of Public Health.

Valenzuela, A., Jr. (2000). Working on the margins: Immigrant day labor characteristics and prospects for employment. The Center for Comparative Immigration Studies, University of California-San Diego.

Valenzuela, A., Jr. (2003). Day labor work. *Annual Review of Psychology*, *29*, 303-333.

Wallerstein, N. (1992). Health and safety education for workers with low-literacy or limited-English skills. *American Journal of Internal Medicine*, *22*(5), 751-65.

doi:10.1300/J187v05n02_08

A Sexual Risk Reduction Intervention for Female Sex Workers in Mexico: Design and Baseline Characteristics

Thomas L. Patterson, PhD
Shirley J. Semple, PhD
Miguel Fraga, MD, MS
Jesus Bucardo, MD, MPH
Adela De la Torre, PhD
Juan Salazar-Reyna, MD

Prisci Orozovich, MPH
Hugo Salvador Staines Orozco, MD
Hortensia Amaro, PhD
Carlos Magis-Rodríguez, MD, MPH
Steffanie A. Strathdee, PhD

Thomas L. Patterson, PhD, is Professor; Shirley J. Semple, PhD, is Project Scientist; Jesus Bucardo, MD, MPH, is Assistant Clinical Professor; Prisci Orozovich, MPH, is Project Manager; and Steffanie A. Strathdee, PhD, is Professor, Harold Simon Chair and Chief of the Division of International Health and Cross-Cultural Medicine, all at the University of California, San Diego, School of Medicine, Department of Psychiatry, La Jolla, CA, USA.

Miguel Fraga, MD, MS, is Professor of Public Health at Facultad de Medicina, Universidad Autónoma de Baja CA, MX.

Adela De la Torre, PhD, is Professor and Director of Chicana/o Studies at University of California, Davis, California, USA.

Juan Salazar-Reyna, MD, is Professor of Medicine at Facultad de Medicina, Universidad Autónoma de Tamaulipas, MX.

Hugo Salvador Staines Orozco, MD, is Chief of Medical Sciences Department at Facultad de Medicina, Universidad Autónoma de Ciudad Juarez, MX.

Hortensia Amaro, PhD, is Distinguished Professor at Bouve College of Health Sciences, Northeastern University, Boston, MA, USA.

Carlos Magis-Rodríguez, MD, MPH, is Director of Research at the National Program for AIDS, México CENSIDA.

[Haworth co-indexing entry note]: "A Sexual Risk Reduction Intervention for Female Sex Workers in Mexico: Design and Baseline Characteristics." Patterson, Thomas L. et al. Co-published simultaneously in *Journal of HIV/AIDS & Social Services* (The Haworth Press, Inc.) Vol. 5, No. 2, 2006, pp. 115-137; and: *Outreach and Care Approaches to HIV/AIDS Along the US-Mexico Border* (ed: Herman Curiel, and Helen Land) The Haworth Press, Inc., 2006, pp. 115-137. Single or multiple copies of this article are available for a fee from The Haworth Document Delivery Service [1-800-HAWORTH, 9:00 a.m. - 5:00 p.m. (EST). E-mail address: docdelivery@haworthpress.com].

Available online at http://jhaso.haworthpress.com
© 2006 by The Haworth Press, Inc. All rights reserved.
doi:10.1300/J187v05n02_09

SUMMARY. Female sex workers (FSWs) 18 or older who reported having unprotected sex with at least one client within the previous month were recruited in Tijuana and Ciudad Juarez, Mexico. After a baseline assessment, participants were randomly assigned to either: (1) Proyecto Comparte Sexo Mas Seguro ("Share Safer Sex"), a theory-based counseling intervention to increase the use of condoms; or (2) time-equivalent voluntary HIV counseling and testing.

Participants had unprotected sex with approximately 27% of clients over the one-month reporting period, and approximately 5% of FSWs in both study conditions tested HIV-seropositive. FSWs in the intervention and comparison conditions showed no significant differences in baseline demographic characteristics, sexual risk behaviors, or HIV serostatus, which indicates that randomization was successful. Future challenges entail participant follow-up and evaluation of intervention effects. doi:10.1300/J187v05n02_09 *[Article copies available for a fee from The Haworth Document Delivery Service: 1-800-HAWORTH. E-mail address: <docdelivery@haworthpress.com> Website: <http://www.HaworthPress.com>* © *2006 by The Haworth Press, Inc. All rights reserved.]*

KEYWORDS. Prostitution, sex work, HIV/AIDS, intervention, sexually transmitted infections, trial

INTRODUCTION

Female sex workers (FSWs) are overrepresented among reported HIV/AIDS cases and other sexually transmitted infections (STIs) in Mexico. However, efforts to change high-risk sexual behavior in this population have been limited. The dramatic increase in HIV/STIs over the past decade, particularly in Mexican cities along the U.S. border, has placed a strain on already limited health resources (Secretaría de Salud, 2001), thereby making prevention programs for FSWs virtually non-existent.

This paper describes the design and baseline sample characteristics for FSWs participating in Proyecto Comparte Sexo Mas Seguro (Share Safer Sex Program [SSS])–a five-year, multisite study that was designed to evaluate the efficacy of a sexual risk reduction counseling program for Mexican FSWs. The four border cities participating in this study are Tijuana, Ciudad Juarez, Nuevo Laredo, and Matamoros. These cities, which range in size from 416,428 to 1.2 million (Secretaría de Turismo, 2000), were selected on the basis of a thriving sex industry, which attracts clients from U.S. border cities. Because of their thriving sex trade, these border cities have some of the highest rates of HIV/STI cases in Mexico (Secretaría de Salud, 2001). A recent modeling exercise suggested that up to one in every 125 persons aged 15-49 in Tijuana may be HIV-infected, and that the number of HIV-infected women in this age group may be as high as 1,296 (Brouwer, Strathdee, & Magis-Rodríguez, in press).

The study design compares the effects of a clinic-based counseling program against a time-equivalent standard counseling condition. Changes in sexual risk behavior will be evaluated among 1800 FSWs (450 per city). Nine hundred FSWs will be randomly assigned to the treatment condition; an equal number will be randomly assigned to the comparison condition. The overall goal of the counseling program is to reduce the number of new HIV/STI infections in this high-risk population and their clients. This project will test the primary hypothesis that a behavioral intervention which integrates a clinical approach with theory-based principles of behavior change is more efficacious in reducing the sexual risk practices of FSWs in border cities of Mexico as compared to a standard HIV testing and counseling condition. We describe the development of Proyecto Comparte Sexo Mas Seguro, loosely translated as "Share Safer Sex," and the characteristics of the baseline sample in the first two Mexican border cities.

METHODS

Theoretical Framework

Proyecto Comparte Sexo Mas Seguro integrates motivational interviewing (MI) and theoretical principles of behavior change. MI is a client-centered, counseling approach that incorporates feedback on current behavior, emphasizes personal responsibility for change, offers clear advice, delineates alternative strategies for changing problem behaviors, promotes counselor empathy and warmth, and reinforces self-efficacy (Miller & Rollnick, 1991). The intervention also incorporates a core set of interrelated constructs derived from Social Cognitive Theory ([SCT]; Bandura, 1986, 1989) and the Theory of Reasoned Action ([TRA]; Fishbein & Ajzen, 1975; Ajzen & Fishbein, 1980).

The elements of SCT include knowledge, self-efficacy, and outcome expectancies. According to SCT, the mechanisms of behavior change involve observation, role modeling, skill performance, positive feedback (practice and rehearsal), and social support (Bandura, 1986, 1989). TRA views intentions as the primary determinant of behavior. Behavioral intentions are determined by the person's attitudes toward performing the behavior and his/her perceptions of social norms associated with the behavior. Personal beliefs regarding the consequences of performing a behavior are seen as shaping attitudes. Perceived social norms, which relate to the individual's perception of others' expectations regarding a particular behavior are also considered a potentially powerful determinant of change (Fishbein & Ajzen, 1975; Ajzen & Fishbein, 1980). Both SCT and TRA view social support as a key element in terms of changing problem behaviors.

Procedures

The design of the study involved the identification of two pairs of comparably-sized cities with random assignment within cities to either the intervention or comparison condition. The first pair of cities was Tijuana and Ciudad Juarez, which are comparably sized (approximately 1.2 million people) and identify maquiladora assembly plants as the main industry (Secretaría de Turismo, 2000). Nuevo Laredo and Matamoros, which identify agriculture and maquiladora assembly plants as their main industry, are also similar in size (approximately 0.5 million people) and were selected as the second pair of cities (Secretaria de Turismo, 2000). The four-city study utilizes a pre-test, post-test, random assignment, treatment-comparison group design (900 women per condition; 450 per city). The methods described in this paper are applicable to all four study sites. However, the baseline sample characteristics are reported for Tijuana and Ciudad Juarez, representing the first pair of border cities to participate in this project, which began in August 2004. Data collection and intervention counseling in Matamoros and Nuevo Laredo are expected to commence in May 2006.

Eligibility Criteria. Potential participants were women (at least 18 years old) who self-identified as FSWs and reported having had unprotected vaginal, oral, or anal sex with a client at least once during the previous month. Exclusion criteria included: (1) consistent use of condoms/dental dam for vaginal, oral and anal sex with all clients during the previous month; (2) employed as a sex worker for less than one month (i.e., to match our period of recall); and (3) under 18 years of age. The latter exclusion criterion was imposed because it is illegal for women under the age of 18 to engage in prostitution in Mexico.

Because of the low frequency of injection drug use among FSWs in these border cities, the intervention did not teach women safer injection practices (e.g., how to clean needles). However, FSWs who reported having ever injected were provided with written Spanish language materials on safer injection practices. Active IDUs were also referred to available drug abuse treatment centers in each city.

FSWs who met all eligibility criteria participated in baseline assessment, safer sex counseling or standard counseling, and six-month follow-up assessment. Women in both the intervention and comparison conditions also received a gynecological examination and laboratory testing (i.e., antibody testing for HIV and specific STIs). Randomization to either the intervention or comparison condition was performed on a weekly basis within each city using a fixed, computer generated randomization scheme (Meinert, 1986).

The interviews and counseling sessions were conducted at a community-based clinic, mobile clinic, private clinic and a government-operated Municipal Medical Clinic. In both Tijuana and Ciudad Juarez, the clinics were located downtown, and within walking distance for the majority of FSWs. Each clinic was equipped with an OB/GYN examination room and several additional counseling rooms. Clinic staff persons in both sites were comprised of one female interviewer and one female counselor, both of whom had prior experience with the study population. The majority of recruitment was conducted through outreach efforts in locations where FSWs were known to work, as well as at the municipal clinic in each participating city. Women were approached in the municipal clinic after they signed up for a doctor's appointment, or in areas where they worked such as bars, streets, brothels and/or massage parlors.

Recruitment. In both cities, recruitment involved venue-based and street outreach approaches. Venue-based recruitment took place at municipal health clinics where FSWs were known to seek health services. At these sites, women were approached after they checked in for their appointment and offered participation. Recruitment via street outreach took place in areas where FSWs worked such as streets, bars, brothels and massage parlors. Trained outreach workers were given five dollar food vouchers for each eligible participant they recruited. In Tijuana, street recruitment also took place using a mobile clinic beginning in August, 2005. The mobile clinic was situated in the "red zone" district where prostitution is tolerated, and was equipped with an examination room and a counseling room.

Data Collection. After providing informed consent, participants were interviewed face-to-face in a private room by clinic staff. Because of low reading level, all materials were administered verbally. The assessment battery required approximately 35 to 40 minutes to complete and covered a range of topics including sexual risk behaviors, working conditions, financial need, victimization and trauma, use of alcohol and illicit drugs, social support, social influence, life experiences, mood, self-esteem, social cognitive factors, socio-demographic characteristics, physical health variables, and psychiatric health variables.

FSWs were paid a total of $30.00 U.S. for completing their baseline assessment, counseling session, and laboratory tests for HIV and specific STIs (gonorrhea, chlamydia, syphilis). All FSWs also received a bag of approximately 100 condoms and lubricant. These incentives were designed to be non-coercive, and to encourage participation in the six-month follow-up assessment. The laboratory tests served two purposes: they provided valuable health information for all participants as well as serving as objective outcome data for this project. Laboratory test results were provided to the FSWs by Municipal Health Clinic staff. When positive test results were obtained, standard notification, counseling, and treatment were provided by the clinic as required by Mexican law.

Description of Proyecto Comparte Sexo Mas Seguro

The development of intervention materials relied heavily upon our pilot work conducted in Tijuana, Mexico (Patterson et al., 2005), and our experience conducting sexual risk reduction interventions in the U.S. In the present study, clinic-based health-care staff were trained to deliver our culturally sensitive sexual risk reduction intervention to FSWs. The content was tailored to the needs, values, beliefs, and behaviors of our target population. The protocol took into account gender and cultural differences in counseling issues, with special consideration given to the ecological validity of our intervention for Latinas. For example, in our pilot study, sex workers indicated that the most important motivator of behavior change was their desire to protect their health so that they might continue to support their children (Patterson et al., 2005). Therefore, we incorporated this important element into our intervention messages. As seen in Table 1, almost all of the women we enrolled had at least one child.

To begin, the counselor asked the participant questions about condom use with clients, including her perceived need to change, possibil-

TABLE 1. Background Characteristics of Female Sex Workers

VARIABLE	SSS	CDC	p-value
Study Site	*(n = 309)*	*(n = 303)*	
Tijuana	137 (44%)	133 (44%)	0.94
Ciudad Juarez	172 (56%)	170 (56%)	
How Recruited?	*(n = 308)*	*(n = 300)*	
Recruiter	120 (39%)	140 (47%)	0.13
Clinic	45 (15%)	44 (15%)	
Study Participant	63 (20%)	52 (17%)	
Other Sex Worker or Friend	45 (15%)	45 (15%)	
Flyer or poster	7 (2%)	0 (0%)	
Other	28 (9%)	19 (6%)	
Age of Participant–Mean (SD)	33 (9.0)	33 (8.0)	0.46
Born in the City of Interview?			
Yes	84 (27%)	91 (30%)	0.47
No	225 (73%)	212 (70%)	
Years Lived in Study Location– Mean (SD)	16.7 (13.1)	17.1 (13.5)	0.75
Marital Status			
Married/Living Together	84 (27%)	79 (26%)	0.78
Separated/Divorced/Widowed/Single	224 (73%)	224 (74%)	
Highest Year of School Completed– Mean (S.D.)	6	6	0.90
# of Children	*(n = 286)*	*(n = 288)*	
0	22 (7%)	15 (5%)	0.42
1-2	126 (41%)	110 (37%)	
3-4	111 (36%)	118 (39%)	
5 or more	49 (16%)	60 (20%)	
Average Age of Children–Mean (SD)	11 (8.0)	11 (7.0)	0.96
Total # of People Living with FSW– Mean (SD)	3 (2.0)	3 (2.0)	0.96
Years Worked in the Sex Trade– Mean (SD)	7.0 (7.4)	6.2 (6.6)	0.13

ity of change, self-efficacy for change, and stated intentions to change. The counselor worked with the participant to increase her awareness of current unsafe behaviors and associated risks (e.g., HIV, STIs, pregnancy). Motivational interviewing techniques (e.g., key questions, reflective listening, summarization, affirmation, and appropriate use of cultural cues) were used to elicit information on the participant's current situation and motivations (Miller & Rollnick, 1991). The goal was to help each woman see her situation clearly and accurately. Helping the individual to understand motivations that underlie her current unsafe behavior with clients was considered a prerequisite step in changing behavior (Miller & Rollnick). For example, we have learned that financial gain is a primary motivation for not using condoms with clients. Other common motivations underlying unsafe sex with clients included the long-term nature of an FSW-client relationship, and discomfort associated with using a condom. As the participant gained insights into her own behavior, she typically began to build motivation for change.

Once awareness of the problem was achieved, the counselor helped the participant discover and understand her motivation for change. This was accomplished by eliciting self-motivated reasons for change and enhancing the participant's self-efficacy for change. Motivations for using condoms with clients were wide ranging (e.g., to avoid diseases and pregnancy, to feel clean, to stay healthy for loved ones, to protect the client, to enjoy sex more, and to save time between clients). Counselors used the "decisional balance" approach to behavior change (Miller & Rollnick, 1991) to help the participant realize that, in most cases, reasons for using condoms with clients strongly outweighed reasons for not using condoms. Once the balance began to shift in favor of positive change, the next step was to help the participant develop a plan of action that best suited her personal situation (Miller & Rollnick). The counselor asked the participant about barriers to condom use, which could include the threat of physical assault or death, rape, loss of clients, and loss of income. The counselor worked with the participant to problem-solve these barriers. The counselor also offered information and suggestions on how to change behavior, and illustrated positive outcomes. The participant was actively involved in the process of problem-solving and was encouraged to come up with solutions. A menu of options was presented. For example, counselors suggested a variety of safer sex options ranging from the use of male and female condoms for vaginal sex, to a variety of harm reduction strategies such as offering the client unprotected oral sex instead of unprotected vaginal sex. According to both MI and SCT, belief in one's ability to bring about change is an important motivator of change (Miller & Rollnick; Bandura, 1986).

The counselor also helped the participant to define achievable goals (e.g., always use a condom for vaginal sex with clients). Once the participant had defined her goals and arrived at a plan of action, the participant and counselor engaged in problem-solving exercises. Alternate choices of behavior and alternative strategies for dealing with the situation were discussed. The counselor aimed to strengthen the woman's commitment to using condoms by exploring ways to make condom use exciting and erotic for the client. The counselor and participant practiced putting a condom on and taking it off a lucite penis model while discussing how to keep the client aroused. The counselor and participant discussed the participant's successes, and the counselor made suggestions for improvement, if necessary. The counseling session took 35 to 40 minutes to complete.

Description of Standard Counseling Session. The comparison condition utilized a modified version of the Centers for Disease Control and Prevention (CDC) revised guidelines for HIV counseling, testing, and referral (CDC, 2001) and materials from Mexico's National Center for AIDS Studies (CENSIDA). The face-to-face standard counseling session took about 35 to 40 minutes to complete. The focus of the counseling session was upon personal risk assessment, cultural identity assessment, and strategies for reducing personal risk. During the personal risk assessment component, the counselor helped the participant identify, understand and acknowledge behaviors and circumstances that put her at risk for contracting HIV and other STIs. The counselor also explored the participant's previous attempts to reduce personal risk, and provided positive reinforcement for positive steps already taken. The counselor also helped the participant to set small, achievable risk-reduction goals and offered concrete suggestions for achieving personal goals (CDC). Basic educational information (e.g., HIV/STI transmission modes) was provided if the woman's level of knowledge was low; however, the primary focus was upon the discussion of transmission risk associated with specific behaviors or activities that were relevant to the participant's personal risk. Lower risk alternatives to risk behavior were promoted (e.g., although oral sex is not risk free, it is associated with lower risk for HIV infection as compared to unprotected vaginal sex).

MEASURES

All measures were translated into Spanish and back-translated into English through the collaborative efforts of Mexican and Latina researchers. Behavioral outcomes assessed in this study included: frequency of unprotected sex with clients and spouse/steady partner; protected sex ratio (number of protected sex acts divided by total number of acts); number of clients; number and type of other sex partners (non-clients); number of partners who inject drugs; number and type of STIs and incidence of HIV/AIDS. We assessed condom use with clients and spouse/steady partner. FSWs also reported the number of times they engaged in vaginal, oral and anal sex without a condom (or dental dam) with clients and their spouse/steady partner during the past month. Additional constructs are described below.

Mechanisms of Change Variables

Knowledge. Our measure of knowledge (Carey & Schroder, 2002) consisted of 18 items, which assessed participants' awareness of the importance of condom use with respect to HIV/STI prevention (e.g., "People who have been infected with HIV quickly show serious signs of being infected"; "A person will not get HIV if she or he is taking antibiotics"). Response categories were True (1) or False (0). Internal consistency alphas range from 0.75 to 0.89, and test-retest reliability range from 0.76 to 0.94 (Carey & Schroder, 2002). Cronbach's alpha using a sample of 81 Tijuana-based FSWs was 0.71.

Self-Efficacy. Our five-item measure of self-efficacy asked participants to indicate the extent to which they were able to use a condom properly with clients. Responses were coded on a 4-point scale (1 = Strongly Disagree to 4 = Strongly Agree). The alpha for this scale was 0.85 (Semple, Patterson, & Grant, 2002).

Outcome Expectancies. Participants responded to five items using a 4-point scale ranging from 1 (Strongly Disagree) to 4 (Strongly Agree). An example of a positive outcome expectancy is: "I believe that condoms will protect me from getting HIV." The alpha for this scale was 0.79 (Semple et al., 2002).

Attitudes Toward AIDS Preventive Acts. Two items were used to measure attitudes toward AIDS preventive acts (Fisher, Kimble-Willcutts, Misovich, & Weinstein, 1998). "My not having (vaginal/oral/anal) intercourse with my clients during the next month would be: very good (5), somewhat good (4), neither good nor bad (3), somewhat bad (2), and very bad (1)"; and "My always using condoms for (vaginal/oral/anal) intercourse with all my clients during the next month would be (response categories above)." Items were asked separately in relation to vaginal, oral, and anal sex. The alpha for this scale was 0.79 (Fisher et al.).

Intentions to Engage in AIDS Preventive Behavior. Intentions were captured by two items: (1) "I intend not to have (vaginal/oral/anal) intercourse with my clients during the next month"; and (2) "I intend to always use condoms for (vaginal/oral/anal) intercourse with all my clients during the next month." Response categories were measured on a 5-point scale (5 = very true; 4 = somewhat true; 3 = neither true nor untrue; 2 = somewhat untrue; 1 = very untrue) (Fisher et al., 1998). Each item was asked separately in relation to vaginal, oral, and anal sex. The alpha for this scale was 0.89.

Perceived Social Norms. Perceived expectations for AIDS prevention behavior were measured by two items: (1) "Most people in my line of work think that I should not have vaginal intercourse with my clients during the next month"; and (2) "Most people in my line of work think that I should always use condoms for vaginal intercourse with all my clients during the next month." Response categories ranged from 1 (very untrue) to 5 (very true) (Fisher et al., 1998). The two items were repeated for oral sex and anal sex with clients. The alpha for this scale was 0.96.

Contextual Factors

Working Conditions were considered to be a multidimensional construct with multiple indicators that include work site (e.g., brothel, street, bar), type of sex worker (e.g., dance hostess, street worker), degree of protection from drunk or aggressive clients, nature of relationship with pimp (if applicable), availability of condoms, earnings, type of sexual services performed, control over selection of clients. An overall rating of work conditions was provided by the participant (1 = very unfavorable) to (5 = very favorable).

Experiences of Abuse were assessed using a measure developed by Strathdee et al. (1997, 1998). This measure assesses three dimensions: non-consensual sex, physical abuse, and emotional abuse. For each dimension, the participant is asked a series of questions: age at first occurrence, age of perpetrator, identity of perpetrator (e.g., client, stepfather), description of abusive activities (e.g., forced unprotected anal intercourse), frequency of abuse, disclosure to others, social support received, and date of most recent incident(s). Current experiences of abuse and childhood history of physical, emotional, and sexual abuse are ascertained along with a variety of global and specific outcomes (e.g., presence/absence of abuse, age of first abuse, frequency of abuse).

Use of Alcohol and Illicit Drugs. FSWs were asked to report their use of alcohol, and a variety of illicit drugs (e.g., marijuana, cocaine, heroin, hallucinogens, methamphetamine, ecstasy). Questions included drug use history and practices (e.g., age at first use of specific drugs, types of drug used and routes of administration within the last month, including inhalation/smoking, ingestion, injection). Among injectors, we collected data on receptive and distributive syringe sharing, frequency of syringe sharing, syringe cleaning and needing help injecting.

Social Factors

Social Support was assessed using a modified version of the Schaefer, Coyne, and Lazarus Inventory (1981). Three dimensions of support were assessed: (1) satisfaction with emotional support; (2) satisfaction with informational support; and (3) network support. The participant was provided with a list of 15 network members. She then rated each person on five items that tap the person's reliability, trustworthiness, caring, confidant qualities, and information provided in relation to safer sex. A 5-point response scale was utilized (1 = not at all to 5 = extremely). Satisfaction with emotional and informational support was averaged across all network members. Network size was defined by the total number of persons rated. Internal consistency reliability for the original scale was 0.95; test-retest reliability was 0.66 (Schaefer et al., 1981).

Social Influence. We assessed the extent to which specific social network members engage in high-risk behaviors. Participants were presented with three categories of individuals: other female sex workers (4 FSWs with whom you have the most contact or feel closest to); pimp; and husband/steady partner. For each of these six individuals, the participant was asked to rate the extent to which this person engaged in the following behaviors: sex with clients without condoms (N/A for pimp and steady); sex with multiple partners without condoms (other than clients for FSWs); drug use before or during sex; alcohol use before or during sex; and intravenous drug use. Ratings were made on a 4-point scale ranging from 1 (not at all) to 4 (very often).

Life Experiences Survey (LES). Participants were presented with a list of events or life changes that are typically experienced in the general population (Sarason, Johnson, & Siegel, 1978). The original list of 47 events was reviewed by a panel of experts from UABC, and modified to enhance cultural sensitivity. Four items were dropped. Three blank spaces permitted the participant to report and rate the occurrence of other events that do not appear on the list. Desirable life experiences and undesirable life experiences were rated separately using a 5-point scale ranging from −2 (extremely negative) to +2 (extremely positive). Positive and negative change scores were summed to create a total change score, which represented all change experienced during the past six months. Test-retest coefficients for the LES total change score were 0.63 and 0.64 in two separate studies (Sarason et al.).

The Sexual Relationship Power Scale was used to assess the relationship between women's perceptions of power and their sexual decision-making. The Sexual Relationship Power Scale (SRPS) assesses the woman's power in intimate relationships as it relates to her role in the couple's approach to decision-making (Pulerwitz, Gortmaker, & DeJong, 2000). The 23-item scale is comprised of two subscales that measure Relationship Control and Decision-Making Dominance within the relationship. Sample items include: "My partner tells me who I can spend time with"; "When my partner and I disagree, he gets his way most of the time." Each of the items was scored on a 4-point scale where 1 = Strongly Agree and 4 = Strongly Disagree. High scores represent high sexual relationship power. The SRPS has good internal consistency reliability and demonstrates both predictive and construct validity. The reliability alpha for the Spanish version scale was 0.88 (Pulerwitz et al.).

Intrapersonal Factors

Depressed Mood was assessed using the depression scale of the Brief Symptom Inventory ([BSI]; Derogatis & Melisaratos, 1983). Cultural sensitivity and appropriateness of scale items were evaluated by researchers at UABC and UCD. All six items in the BSI depression scale were judged as appropriate for use with the target population. The internal consistency alpha for the depression scale was .84 in this sample.

Self-Esteem. Self-esteem is an element of self-concept that refers to the regard in which one holds oneself (Rosenberg, 1965). The Rosenberg self-esteem scale consists of eight items measured on a 4-point scale ranging from 1 (Strongly Disagree) to 4 (Strongly Agree). Sample items include: "I feel that I have a number of good qualities"; "I wish I could have more respect for myself"; and "On the whole, I am satisfied with myself." The self-esteem scale has good test-retest reliability, as well as construct validity (Grossman, Wirt, & Davids, 1985; Orshan, 1999).

Background Characteristics

Financial Need was assessed by five items that asked about the participant's earnings from sex work, earnings from other sources of work, number of people who are financial dependents, and the nature of relationship with financial dependents. An overall rating of financial need was also obtained, ranging from 1 (extremely bad) to 5 (extremely good).

Occupational Choice. Discussion of occupational choice and sexuality preference is an emerging concept within the feminist theory discourse on prostitution. The implications of this debate are linked to assessment of interpretations of agency or power that FSWs may have in the workplace. We used a measure of occupational choice that asked the following question, "Did any of the following influence you to be a sex worker?" A list of 23 items was presented (e.g., pay the rent, utilities, food; pays better than other work). A dichotomous response category was utilized (1 = Yes, 0 = No). Summary scores ranged from 0 to 23.

Acculturation was assessed using the Acculturation Rating Scale for Mexican Americans-II (ARSMA), developed by Cuellar, Arnold, and Maldonado (1995). The ARSMA-II consists of 12 items that explore processes associated with cultural patterning and social integration by examining language familiarity and usage, ethnic interaction, ethnic pride and identity, cultural heritage, and generational proximity. Sample items include: "I enjoy English language movies" and "My thinking is done in the English language." Response categories range from 1 (Not at all) to 5 (Extremely often or almost always). Summary scores ranged from 12 to 60.

Biologic Assays

Serology was performed at baseline and six-month follow-up on a venipuncture specimen to test for syphilis and to ascertain the HIV serostatus of participants. The blood draw and testing took place at the various clinics. FSWs also received a gynecological exam and obtained a cervical specimen to test for chlamydia and gonorrhea. Other STIs were assessed by self-report.

RESULTS

Sample Characteristics. A total of 641 FSWs were screened for eligibility, of whom 612 (95.5%) met screening eligibility criteria and were enrolled. Of these, 270 were recruited in Tijuana, 137 of whom were randomized to the intervention (denoted SSS) and 133 to the comparison condition (denoted CDC). An additional 342 women were recruited in Ciudad Juarez and randomized to either SSS (N = 172) or CDC (N =

170). The majority of participants in both sites were recruited through referrals from other participants, with street outreach being the second most common method of recruitment.

As shown in Table 1, there were no significant demographic differences between the intervention and comparison conditions. The average age of participants in both conditions was 33 years, and women averaged 6th grade education or less. Most were born in Mexican cities other than where they were recruited, and had lived in their recruitment city for an average of 13 years. About a quarter of the women were married or living with a partner. More than 90% had children who were an average of 11 years old.

Sexual Risk Behavior with Clients. By design, all women reported having engaged in unprotected sex with at least one client during the past month. There were no significant differences in sexual behaviors between those randomized to the SSS or CDC conditions. All women reported having unprotected vaginal sex, 50% reported unprotected oral sex, and 12% unprotected anal sex with clients. Fifty-two percent reported never or sometimes using condoms for vaginal sex, with the remainder reporting sometimes using a condom. However, none of the women were able to produce a condom at the time of the interview. Women reported having an average of 52 (S.D. $+/-57$) clients in the past month.

Participants were also asked about their specific sexual behaviors with regular versus non-regular clients. Regular clients were defined as "men who come back to you for repeat visits/men that you have an ongoing relationship with over time." Non-regular clients were defined as "men who do not come back to you for regular visits/men that you have seen only once or twice." FSWs in the intervention and comparison conditions did not differ in terms of their sexual risk behaviors with regular and non-regular partners as reported for the previous month. FSWs in both conditions reported approximately six regular partners and had an average of eight unprotected vaginal sex acts, one unprotected anal sex act, and three unprotected oral sex acts with regular partners. Moreover, FSWs in the intervention and comparison conditions reported approximately 45 non-regular clients and had an average of 13 acts of unprotected vaginal sex, one unprotected anal sex act, and five unprotected oral sex acts with non-regular partners. These findings appear in Table 2.

Sexual Risk Behaviors with Spouse/Steady Partner. As shown in Table 2, approximately 36% of FSWs in both conditions reported having a

TABLE 2. Sexual Risk Behaviors with Clients and Spouse/Steady Partner

SEXUAL BEHAVIOR WITH:				
ALL CLIENTS	Category/ Statistics	SSS	CDC	p-value
Unprotected vaginal sex in past month	Yes	309 (100%)	303 (100%)	1.0
	No	0 (0%)	0 (0%)	
Unprotected oral sex in past month	Yes	149 (48%)	152 (50%)	0.68
	No	160 (52%)	151 (50%)	
Unprotected anal sex in past month	Yes	37 (12%)	34 (11%)	0.80
	No	272 (88%)	269 (89%)	
REGULAR CLIENTS	Category/ Statistics	SSS	CDC	p-value
Have one or more regular clients	Yes	290 (94%)	283 (93%)	0.82
	No	19 (6%)	20 (7%)	
# of regular clients	Mean (SD)	6 (8.0)	5 (8.0)	0.08
# vaginal sex acts in past month	Mean (SD)	20 (21.0)	16 (16.0)	0.06
# vaginal sex using condoms in past month	Mean (SD)	11 (14)	9 (13)	0.06
# anal sex in past month	Mean (SD)	1 (2)	1 (6)	0.50
# anal sex using condoms in past month	Mean (SD)	0 (1)	0 (1)	0.17
# oral sex in past month	Mean (SD)	7 (14)	5 (8)	0.33
# oral sex using condoms in past month	Mean (SD)	4 (10)	3 (6)	0.55
NON-REGULAR CLIENTS	Statistics	SSS	CDC	p-value
# of non-regular clients	Mean (SD)	46 (53)	44 (52)	0.65
# vaginal sex in past month	Mean (SD)	52 (57)	46 (56)	0.08
# vaginal sex using condoms in past month	Mean (SD)	38 (47)	34 (48)	0.13
# anal sex in past month	Mean (SD)	1 (3)	1 (5)	0.43
# anal sex using condoms in past month	Mean (SD)	0 (3)	0 (2)	0.61
# oral sex in past month	Mean (SD)	18 (42)	12 (30)	0.85
# oral sex using condoms in past month	Mean (SD)	12 (34)	8 (22)	0.53
# of condoms in FSW's possession	Mean (SD)	0 (2)	0 (1)	0.74
SPOUSE OR STEADY PARTNER	Category/ Statistics	SSS	CDC	p-value
Have spouse or steady partner	Yes	113 (37%)	106 (35%)	0.74
	No	196 (63%)	197 (65%)	
# vaginal sex in past month	Mean (SD)	14 (18)	11 (10)	0.47
# vaginal sex in past month using a condom	Mean (SD)	1 (3)	1 (2)	0.50
# anal sex in past month	Mean (SD)	1 (4)	1 (4)	0.90
# anal sex in past month using a condom	Mean (SD)	0 (1)	0 (1)	0.20
# oral sex in past month	Mean (SD)	6 (13)	5 (8)	0.92
# oral sex in past month using a condom	Mean (SD)	1 (4)	0 (1)	0.88

spouse or steady partner. There were no differences between the two conditions in terms of the mean number of unprotected vaginal, anal, or oral sex acts. Vaginal sex with spouse/steady partner was almost always unprotected. On average, participants in both conditions reported 12 unprotected vaginal sex acts in a one-month period. Anal sex with a spouse/steady partner was rarely reported. The average number of unprotected anal sex acts was one in both groups. With respect to oral sex, the average number of unprotected acts with a spouse/steady partner was five during the past month.

Drug and Alcohol Risk Behaviors. We examined baseline differences between intervention and comparison subjects in terms of three drug and alcohol risk behaviors. Participants in the intervention and comparison conditions did not differ in terms of their use of alcohol or illicit drugs before having sex with a client as assessed over the previous month. In both conditions, approximately 23% used alcohol "Often" or "Always" before having sex with clients. Moreover, approximately 12% of FSWs in both groups used illicit drugs "Often" or "Always" before having sex with clients. Participants were also asked if they had ever injected drugs. There were no differences between the two groups in terms of the percentage who responded affirmatively to this question. Approximately 17% of FSWs in both conditions reported having injected drugs at least once in their lifetime. Findings are presented in Table 3.

HIV Serostatus from Lab Tests and Self-Report. As shown in Table 4, laboratory results for HIV serostatus using the Western Blot Confirmation Method revealed an HIV-positive serostatus rate of approximately 5% in both the intervention and comparison conditions. Among participants who self-reported their HIV serostatus, the HIV-positive serostatus rate was less than 2% in both groups, indicating a discrepancy between actual and reported rates. There were no significant differences in self-report of HIV serostatus between the intervention and comparison conditions. Prior to enrollment in our study, only 49% had ever had an HIV test.

This research is a work in process. The wide scope of data collected for this study, and various stages of data reduction have limited reporting and analysis of all the variables available for this report. Results from analysis of some of the variables from instruments described above will be available in the near future. It is hoped forthcoming articles will touch upon some of the following themes in which data has been collected but is not yet ready for description or analysis in this paper:

TABLE 3. Drug and Alcohol Use Risk Behaviors

VARIABLE	SSS	CDC	p-value
Used alcohol before sex with client in past month			
Never	124 (41%)	102 (35%)	0.06
Sometimes	114 (38%)	116 (40%)	
Often	28 (9%)	27 (9%)	
Always	34 (11%)	47 (16%)	
Used illegal drugs before sex with client in past month			
Never	232 (75%)	202 (67%)	0.11
Sometimes	44 (14%)	62 (20%)	
Often	10 (3%)	17 (6%)	
Always	22 (7%)	22 (7%)	
Ever injected drugs?			
No	259 (84%)	248 (82%)	0.52
Yes	49 (16%)	55 (18%)	

TABLE 4. HIV Serostatus from Laboratory Test and Self-Report

VARIABLE	SSS	CDC	p-value
Baseline result of Western Blot	*(n = 309)*	*(n = 302)*	
Positive	16 (5.2%)	16 (5.3%)	0.08
Negative	10 (3.2%)	2 (0.66%)	
Last HIV test result (self-reported)	*(n = 162)*	*(n = 158)*	
Positive	3 (2%)	1 (1%)	0.38
Negative	151 (93%)	148 (94%)	
Didn't understand results	0 (0%)	2 (1%)	
Never received results	8 (5%)	7 (4%)	

- Mechanisms of change (i.e., knowledge, self-efficacy, outcome expectancy, attitudes, intentions, and perceived social norms);
- Contextual factors (i.e., working conditions and experiences of abuse);
- Social factors (i.e., social support, social influence, life experiences survey, and sexual relationship power scale);
- Intra-personal factors (i.e., depression and self-esteem);

• Background characteristics (i.e., financial need, occupational choice, and acculturation); and biological tests for STDs.

DISCUSSION

Proyecto Comparte Sexo Mas Seguro is a brief safer-sex intervention designed specifically for female sex workers in Mexican border cities. This theory-based intervention was based on social cognitive theory with elements of motivational interviewing (MI). The intervention was developed with the assistance of Latina women, which ensured that the intervention was both practical and culturally appropriate for this population. The integration of MI into our intervention was considered important because it allows women to identify factors that motivate them to practice safer sex with clients. For example, the fact that 90% of these FSWs had at least one child suggests that promoting one's health to enable one to continue parenting may be a powerful motivator of behavior change, as suggested by our pilot work (Patterson et al., 2005). Social service providers should be aware of the high proportion of FSWs who have children since both are likely to require specialized services such as child care, educational and health promotion.

As the baseline results indicate, the Proyecto Comparte Sexo Mas Seguro baseline data was gathered from a diverse sample of FSWs from two Mexican border cities (i.e., Tijuana and Ciudad Juarez). By design, all women reported unprotected sex with at least one client in the previous month, with an average of nearly two clients per day. Despite this relatively low level of transactional sex, unprotected sex was reported with approximately one in four clients. This suggests that there is a great need for interventions designed to reduce such high-risk behavior. Self-reported rates of HIV were low as compared to actual rates as determined by laboratory tests. This could be due to infrequent testing for HIV, denial, or socially desirable responses. Future studies of FSWs should rely on objective measures of HIV serostatus, which are likely to be higher than those reported by research participants. Additionally, since only half of the FSWs in this study had ever had an HIV test, the role of social service providers and "promotoras" [outreach workers] should be to promote awareness of HIV and the need for regular testing and counseling.

It would be desirable to design a behavioral intervention with multiple sessions that took into account other issues facing this population, such as poverty, substance use, and other environmental and structural factors. Indeed, in an earlier report from this study, we found high levels of illicit drug use in this population, including injection drug use (Patterson et al., in press). However, as might be expected in such a re-source-poor environment with such a mobile population, our participant sex workers indicated a preference for brief interventions that would not be overly burdensome (Patterson et al., 2005). In other populations, such as injection drug users who are not also sex workers, financial in-centives are often enough to sustain long-term participation. By con-trast, sex workers can earn more on the street than they can from an intervention. For that very reason, a longer intervention might impede efforts at recruitment and retention of sex workers.

The majority of FSWs had both regular and non-regular clients. The pattern of sexual risk behavior was similar for both types of clients. Vaginal sex was the most commonly reported sex act. Oral sex occurred less frequently and anal sex was rarely reported. On average, women re-ported having unprotected vaginal sex with clients about one-third of the time. This suggests that FSWs have access to condoms and are will-ing to use them with both regular and non-regular clients. More research is needed to enhance our understanding of the barriers to condom use with clients and to determine if barriers differ according to regular and non-regular client types. Sexual risk behaviors with spouses and steady partners was almost always unprotected. This finding is consistent with previous studies of the sexual practices of Latinas residing in Mexico and immigrant Latinas in the United States (Nyamathi, Bennett, Leake, Lewis, & Flaskerud, 1993).

In terms of substance use, a substantial proportion of women re-ported frequently using alcohol prior to having sex with clients. This may reflect the use of alcohol as a coping strategy. High levels of alco-hol use have been reported in studies of FSWs in both developed and underdeveloped countries (de Graaf, Vanwesenbeeck, van Zessen, Straver, & Visser, 1995; El-Bassel, Simoni, Cooper, Gilbert, & Schilling, 2001; Peltzer, Seoka, & Raphala, 2004; Persaud, Klaskala, Tewari, Shultz, & Baum, 1999). In one study of FSWs in Papua New Guinea, al-cohol use was cited as a common reason for not using condoms with cli-ents at all times (Mgone et al., 2002). Nearly one-fifth of the FSWs in both Tijuana and Ciudad Juarez reported having injected drugs at least once in their lifetime, which is also cause for concern. In a recent study, Viani and colleagues (2005) found that the prevalence of HIV among pregnant women in Tijuana was 1% which was linked to drug use. Other studies suggest that injection drug use and associated risk behav-iors are on the rise in Tijuana and Ciudad Juarez (Bucardo et al., 2005;

Strathdee et al., 2005). This social phenomenon places FSWs who inject drugs at high risk of acquiring HIV and other blood borne infections. There is therefore a growing need for social service providers to promote drug abuse treatment and help link FSWs who use drugs to such services, when available.

A rigorous evaluation of the Proyecto Comparte Sexo Mas Seguro clinical trial will provide valuable information on the efficacy of this intervention. The brief nature of the counseling session suggests that it can be practically implemented in diverse community settings. If proven to be efficacious, widespread implementation of this tailored sexual risk reduction intervention could help to reduce the number of new cases of HIV and other STIs among female sex workers and their clients in Mexico border cities.

AUTHOR NOTE

Address correspondence to: Thomas L. Patterson, PhD, Department of Psychiatry (0680), University of California, San Diego, 9500 Gilman Drive, La Jolla, CA 92093-0680 (E-mail: tpatterson@ucsd.edu).

The authors respectfully acknowledge the participation of all women in this study, and especially thank study staff for making this work possible. They also thank Brian Kelly for editorial assistance and Dr. Willo Pequegnat at the National Institute of Mental Health for her support and encouragement. Support for this research was provided through NIMH grant 5 R01 MH65849, 5 R01 MH62554-Supp, and UCSD Center for AIDS Research grant P30 AI36214-06.

REFERENCES

Ajzen, I., & Fishbein, M. (1980). *Understanding attitudes and predicting social behavior.* Englewood Cliffs, NJ: Prentice-Hall.

Bandura, A. (1986). *Social foundations of thought and action: A social cognitive theory.* Englewood Cliffs, NJ: Prentice-Hall.

Bandura, A. (1989). Perceived self-efficacy. In V. Mays, G. Albee, & S. Schneider (Eds.), *Primary prevention of AIDS: Psychological approaches* (pp. 128-141). Newbury Park, CA: Sage.

Brouwer, K. C., Strathdee, S. A., & Magis-Rodriguez, C. (in press). Estimated numbers of men and women infected with HIV/AIDS in Tijuana, Mexico. *Journal of Urban Health.*

Bucardo, J., Brouwer, K. C., Fraga, M., Perez, S. G., Patterson, T. L., & Strathdee, S. A. (2005). Historical trends in the production and consumption of illicit drugs in Mexico: Implications for the prevention of blood borne infections. *Drug and Alcohol Dependence, 79,* 281-293.

Carey, M. P., & Schroder, K. E. (2002). Development and psychometric evaluation of the brief HIV knowledge questionnaire (HIV-KQ-18). *AIDS Education and Prevention, 14*, 172-182.

Centers for Disease Control and Prevention (2001). *Revised guidelines for HIV counseling, testing, and referral.* Atlanta: CDC.

Cuellar, I., Arnold, B., & Maldonado, R. (1995). Acculturation Rating Scale for Mexican Americans-II: A revision of the original ARSMA Scale. *Hispanic Journal of Behavioral Sciences, 17*, 275-304.

de Graaf, R., Vanwesenbeeck, I., van Zessen, G., Straver, C. J., & Visser, J. H. (1995). Alcohol and drug use in heterosexual and homosexual prostitution, and its relation to protection behaviour. *AIDS Care, 7*, 35-47.

Derogatis, L. R., & Melisaratos, N. (1983). The Brief Symptom Inventory: An introductory report. *Psychological Medicine, 13*, 595-605.

El-Bassel, N., Simoni, J. M., Cooper, D. K., Gilbert, L., & Schilling, R. F. (2001). Sex trading and psychological distress among women on methadone. *Psychology of Addictive Behaviors, 15*, 177-184.

Fishbein, M., & Ajzen, I. (1975). *Belief, attitude, intention, and behavior: An introduction to theory and research.* Reading, MA: Addison-Wesley.

Fisher, J. D., Kimble-Willcutts, D. L., Misovich, S. J., & Weinstein, B. (1998). Dynamics of sexual risk behavior in HIV-infected men who have sex with men. *AIDS and Behavior, 2,* 101-113.

Grossman, B., Wirt, R., & Davids, A. (1985). Self-esteem, ethnic identity, and behavioral adjustment among Anglo and Chicano adolescents in West Texas. *Journal of Adolescence, 8*, 57-68.

Meinert, C. L. (1986). *Clinical trials: Design, conduct, and analysis.* New York: Oxford University Press.

Mgone, C. S., Passey, M. E., Anang, J., Peter, W., Lupiwa, T., Russell, D. M. et al. (2002). Human immunodeficiency virus and other sexually transmitted infections among female sex workers in two major cities in Papua New Guinea. *Sexually Transmitted Diseases, 29*, 265-270.

Miller, W. R., & Rollnick, S. (1991). *Motivational interviewing: Preparing people to change addictive behavior.* New York: The Guilford Press.

Nyamathi, A., Bennett, C., Leake, B., Lewis, C., & Flaskerud, J. (1993). AIDS-related knowledge, perceptions, and behaviors among impoverished minority women. *American Journal of Public Health, 83*, 65-71.

Orshan, S. A. (1999). Acculturation, perceived social support, self-esteem, and pregnancy status among Dominican adolescents. *Health Care for Women International, 20*, 245-247.

Patterson, T. L., Semple, S. J., Fraga, M., Bucardo, J., Davila-Fraga, W., & Strathdee, S. (2005). An HIV-prevention intervention for sex workers in Tijuana, Mexico: A pilot study. *Hispanic Journal of Behavioral Sciences, 27*, 82-100.

Patterson, T. L., Semple, S. J., Fraga, M., Bucardo, J., De la Torre, A., Salazar, J. et al. (in press). Comparison of sexual and drug use behaviors between female sex workers in Tijuana and Cuidad Juarez, Mexico. *Substance Use and Misuse.*

Peltzer, K., Seoka, P., & Raphala, S. (2004). Characteristics of female sex workers and their HIV/AIDS/STI knowledge, attitudes and behaviour in semi-urban areas in South Africa. *Curationis, 27,* 4-11.

Persaud, N. E., Klaskala, W., Tewari, T., Shultz, J., & Baum, M. (1999). Drug use and syphilis: Co-factors for HIV transmission among commercial sex workers in Guyana. *West Indian Medical Journal, 48,* 52-56.

Pulerwitz, J., Gortmaker, S. L., & DeJong, W. (2000, April). Measuring sexual relationship power in HIV/STD research. *Sex Roles: A Journal of Research,* 637-660.

Rosenberg, M. (1965). *Society and the adolescent self-image.* Princeton, NJ: Princeton University Press.

Sarason, I., Johnson, J., & Siegel, J. (1978). Assessing the impact of life changes: Development of the Life Experiences Survey. *Journal of Consulting and Clinical Psychology, 46,* 932-946.

Schaefer, C., Coyne, J. C., & Lazarus, R. (1981). The health-related functions of social support. *Journal of Behavioral Medicine, 4,* 381-406.

Secretaría de Salud y Asistencia, Instituto Nacional de Salud Pública, Consejo Nacional para la Prevención y Control del SIDA (2001, Mayo). *Reporte Anual de VIAH/SIDA-2000* [Annual Report on HIV/AIDS]. Mexico, D.F. [Mexico City].

Secretaría de Turismo (SECTUR), Gobierno Federal de Mexico (2000, Julio). *Reporte: Actividad Fronteriza* [Report: Border Activity]. Mexico, D.F. [Mexico City].

Semple, S. J., Patterson, T. L., & Grant, I. (2002). Gender differences in the sexual risk practices of HIV + heterosexual men and women. *AIDS and Behavior, 6,* 45-54.

Strathdee, S. A., Davila-Fraga, W., Case, P., Firestone, M., Brouwer, K. C., Perez, S. G. et al. (2005). "Vivo para consumirla y la consumo para vivir" ["I live to inject it and I inject it to live"]: High risk injection behaviors in Tijuana, Mexico. *Journal of Urban Health, 82*(3 Suppl 4), iv58-73.

Strathdee, S. A., Hogg, R. S., Martindale, S. L., Cornelisse, P. G. A., Craib, K. J. P., Montaner, J. S. G. et al. (1998). Determinants of sexual risktaking among young HIV-negative gay men. *Journal of Acquired Immune Deficiency Syndromes and Human Retrovirology, 19,* 61-66.

Strathdee, S. A., Patrick, D. M., Archibald, C. P., Ofner, M., Cornelisse, P. G. A., Rekart, M. L. et al. (1997). Social determinants predict needle sharing behaviour among injection drug users in Vancouver, Canada. *Addiction, 92,* 1339-1347.

Viani, R. M., Araneta, M. R. G., Ruiz-Calderon, J., Hubbard, P., Lopez, G., Chacoon-Cruz, E. et al. (2005). Perinatal HIV counseling and rapid testing in Tijuana, Baja California, Mexico. *Journal of Acquired Immune Deficiency Syndromes, 41,* 87-92.

doi:10.1300/J187v05n02_09

A Transcultural Case Management Model for HIV/AIDS Care and Prevention

Rebeca L. Ramos, MPH
João B. Ferreira-Pinto, PhD

SUMMARY. The Transcultural Case Management (TCM) intervention utilizing community health-care workers–*Promotores*–was designed to increase adherence to Highly Active Anti-Retroviral Therapy (HAART) treatment. The TCM model was also expected to help reduce the use of

Rebeca L. Ramos, MPH, is Technical Director at the United States-México Border Health Association.

João B. Ferreira-Pinto, PhD, is Senior Researcher at the Border Planning and Evaluation Group.

Address correspondence to: João B. Ferreira-Pinto, PhD, Senior Researcher, Border Planning and Evaluation Group, 505 Granada, El Paso, TX 79912 (E-mail: joao@bpegroup.org) or Rebeca L. Ramos, MPH, Technical Director of the US Mexico Border Health Association (E-mail: rebeca@utep.edu).

The authors would like to thank the United States-México Border Health Association (USMBHA), the Centers for Disease Control and Prevention (CDC), and the organizations that participated in discussions of the potential application of the findings and supported the dissemination of the program. Also, they give special thanks to the participating Health Management Alliances (HMAs) of New Mexico, and most importantly to the Promotores, who have provided the impetus for the program and continue to provide care and prevention services to Hispanic populations in New Mexico and throughout the United States.

The implementation and data collection on the TCM model was funded by grant # 25-P-91070/6-01 from the Centers for Medicare and Medicaid Services (CMS).

[Haworth co-indexing entry note]: "A Transcultural Case Management Model for HIV/AIDS Care and Prevention." Ramos, Rebeca L., and João B. Ferreira-Pinto. Co-published simultaneously in *Journal of HIV/AIDS & Social Services* (The Haworth Press, Inc.) Vol. 5, No. 2, 2006, pp. 139-157; and: *Outreach and Care Approaches to HIV/AIDS Along the US-Mexico Border* (ed: Herman Curiel, and Helen Land) The Haworth Press, Inc., 2006, pp. 139-157. Single or multiple copies of this article are available for a fee from The Haworth Document Delivery Service [1-800-HAWORTH, 9:00 a.m. - 5:00 p.m. (EST). E-mail address: docdelivery@haworthpress.com].

Available online at http://jhaso.haworthpress.com
© 2006 by The Haworth Press, Inc. All rights reserved.
doi:10.1300/J187v05n02_10

hospital emergency rooms, the number of hospitalization days, and consequently to lower treatment costs among Hispanic HIV-positive male patients.

The intervention results, although not statistically significant because of a higher than expected attrition rate and difficulties in accessing patients for follow-up, were in the expected direction. Furthermore, the self-reported quality of life of the patients increased by the development of social networks among patients and by an increased sense of self-reliance and empowerment. Problems encountered in fulfilling the goals of the research protocol, and recommendations on how to improve research in HIV care organizations are also discussed. doi:10.1300/J187v05n02_10

[Article copies available for a fee from The Haworth Document Delivery Service: 1-800-HAWORTH. E-mail address: <docdelivery@haworthpress.com> Website: <http://www.HaworthPress.com> © 2006 by The Haworth Press, Inc. All rights reserved.]

KEYWORDS. Promotores, immigrants, Hispanic, Latinos, HIV/AIDS, US-Mexico border, HIV health care

INTRODUCTION

Highly Active Anti-Retroviral Therapy (HAART) regimens, incorporating recently developed drugs, have been steadily moving acute care HIV treatment towards a chronic disease model, and HIV patients managed under these improved drug regimens have the potential of attaining the anticipated lifespan of non-HIV people their own age (Schackman et al., 2002). The survival rate among HIV patients will continue to increase, as will the cohort of HIV-seropositive patients requiring a lifelong supply of medications and specialized medical attention needed to monitor drug regimens calibrated to each patient's changing therapeutic needs (Murphy et al., 2001). The Centers for Medicare and Medicaid Services (CMS), the main governmental agency financing the free distribution of HAART medicines and services, needs to develop mechanisms to contain growing treatment costs if it is to remain solvent (Palella et al., 1998; Hellinger, 1998). Although cost of medications included in a typical HAART regimen is expected to decrease over time and when patents expire and generic substitutes become available, in the end, the cost of medical attention is left as the main target for cost-savings. One of the proposed strategies to decrease the cost of medical care is to shift medical attention to less costly providers, such as nurse practitioners and physician assistants (Bozzette et al., 2001). Another strategy, which is examined in detail in this article, is to decrease the number of crises and emergency treatment episodes and their associated hospitalization costs. Such factors may be avoided by early detection.

COST-SAVING STRATEGIES

Effective strategies to deal with medical emergencies include early initiation of medical care at the onset of even minor health problems, and monitoring the adherence to prescribed HAART regimens, which jointly comprise the most promising cost-saving strategy in HIV/AIDS care.

Reasons for patients' non-adherence to HAART regimens are varied and include patient-related factors, such as substance and alcohol abuse, homelessness, mental illness, and the low levels of health literacy about treatments exhibited by most patients (Chesney, 2000). The health-care professional-patient relationship is also important for adherence to HAART regimens, and Krantz (2003) reports that those patients who perceived their provider as more accessible had better adherence to anti-retroviral regimens. Cultural and language differences between patients and providers are also barriers to adherence (Murphy, Roberts, Hoffman, Molina, & Lu, 2003). Many providers do not take into consideration that oftentimes the prescribed treatment is contrary to the patient's belief system, and when dealing with patients with limited English proficiency, interpreters are not employed effectively (Ramos & Ferreira-Pinto, 2002). Adherence is also negatively affected by the complexity of the treatment regimen. The number of medications, dietary restrictions, dosing schedules, medication side effects, and the amount of distress such medications cause significantly hinder the ability to follow the prescribed regimen effectively (McDonnell et al., 2003).

The lack of adherence to medications is a major cause of avoidable emergency room visits. Compounding the problem is lack of knowledge of the signs of an impending medical emergency; thus, many fail to obtain medical care that could prevent a medical crisis at the onset.

In light of these pressing needs, the present TCM intervention was designed to improve patients' adherence to treatment and acceptance of the need for early detection and treatment of medical conditions, by seeking the help of health-care providers at the onset of even minor ailments. The main research goal of the study was to determine if improvements in these two factors would significantly decrease the number of visits to hospital emergency rooms and reduce hospitalization days. The intervention was also designed to be cost-effective and easily replicable, and also to improve the patients' self-reliance and overall quality of life.

The intervention described herein is labeled the Transcultural Case Management (TCM) model. The model is transcultural, insofar as it serves to bridge the differences between providers working within the medical paradigms of the dominant culture and patients who may belong to another culture and may have a different view of acceptable medical procedures.

The TCM is based on a version of case management that employs lay health-care workers, henceforth referred to as *Promotores*. Such workers foster better communications between health providers and patients by serving as liaisons and offer counsel to patients on how to better manage HIV disease. It is expected that this increased communication will result in better reporting of anomalous physical or mental conditions that could indicate the onset of an opportunistic infection, or the beginning of a non-adherence episode, either of which could result in costly medical emergencies and increased suffering for patients.

ORIGINS OF THE TCM MODEL

The TCM model is based on the lessons learned from Promovisión, a project based on the use of Promotores designed to facilitate access to health services to HIV+ Latinos. The use of Promotores is central to the model and is based on their success in a number of health-care and prevention domains. Traditionally, Promotores have acted as prevention outreach workers among marginalized populations in Africa (Chabot, 1987), Asia (Wang, 1975), and Latin America (Stasiak, 1991). In the U.S., they have provided outreach to underserved minority populations in the Southwest since the 1980s (Giblin, 1989; Warrick, Wood, Meister, & de Zapien, 1992). The key to Promotores' success in the U.S. is their knowledge of the nuances of language and culture so necessary for the adaptation and delivery of prevention messages to Hispanic populations (Scholl, 1985). The Promovisión project expanded this traditional outreach work to include a liaison component between medical providers and HIV clients to help clarify to case managers the reasons for patients' demands. In addition, Promotores helped clients understand the financial and personnel limitations that hinder the case manager's ability to provide requested services (Ramos, Hernandez, Ferreira-Pinto, Ortiz, & Gallegos, 2006). This component was incorporated into the TCM project to extend the breadth of the patients' contacts with medical care providers and to facilitate early treatment and adherence to medications and treatment components.

One of the findings of the original Promovisión project that became central to the expansion of the TCM model was the importance of a patient's perception of the level of the care necessary to provide a successful outcome of HIV treatment. Research has shown that, regardless of the expertise of caregivers, the greater the amount of personal attention HIV patients receive, the better is their general well-being and medical outcome (Fleishman, 1997). High level of material and affective support from a tight social network is also shown to increase the immune system's response to outside stressors thus preventing the onset of infirmities in HIV patients (Friedland, Renwick, & Mccoll, 1996; Leserman et al., 2000). Additionally, increased contact between patients and providers both positively influences adherence to treatment, and appears to be the most important factor in improved health outcomes (Markson, Houchens, Fanning, & Turner, 1998).

Freirian pedagogical principles, applied to health education, were at the core of the Promovisión project and were replicated in the TCM model. Paulo Freire (1970) suggests that the role of any educator is to study the heuristic devices that learners employ to understand and navigate their world, and then to codify them into culturally relevant themes in order to help learners better understand new concepts. Applying these principles to the TCM model, Promotores first had to learn from HIV patients what barriers they felt were impeding them from taking better care of their health, and what would empower patients to manage better the physical and psychological demands of their disease.

PROMOTORES AND THE TCM MODEL

Being the core element in the TCM model, the selection of appropriate Promotores was crucial to the successful implementation of this model. For this study, Promotores were recruited among HIV patients in Health Maintenance Alliance (HMA) HIV clinics in New Mexico (HMA, 2004). The selection was a joint decision of the HMA management and the research team, and based on the recruited patient's bilingual/bicultural skills, ethnic identification with the target population, communication skills, and familiarity with the medical and case management procedures of the HMA staff to which he or she would be assigned. After being selected, the Promotores were trained in the skills necessary to provide HIV case management to Hispanic patients. Hands-on activities and experiential learning were emphasized during the training, as were skills necessary to conduct preliminary needs assessments. Under the tutelage and supervision of an experienced HMA case manager they were taught the procedures to refer patients to services for which the patients qualified. To increase their expertise and to better serve their clients, Promotores periodically attended training on new HIV treatments, fraud detection, clinical trials enrollment procedures, legal rights and responsibilities, alternative and complementary therapies, nutrition, and other related subjects.

Because they were HMA patients themselves, the Promotores were known by the research target patients and perceived by them as having a better understanding of the problems related to their HIV status. In addition, by having increased contact with patients, Promotores could obtain timely information from patients and their support network about the patients' health status. In addition, because of their more frequent contact with patients, Promotores were more readily able to detect health-related problems than could the case managers, who mostly had brief meetings with patients on a monthly basis. It was expected that information gathered about patients and discussed with case managers would inform the practical advice provided by Promotores, and patients would learn from the Promotores about how to monitor their own health status more closely and to obtain more readily the medical and social services needed to stay healthy, and have a better overall quality of life.

In the TCM model, the Promotore is primarily a liaison between patients and case managers and acts as an interpreter explaining to patients the instructions given by case managers about medical and social services. The Promotore also interprets to case managers the problems patients have with medical regimens, medications and access to social services and, importantly, they propose solutions to these problems. In this role, the Promotore may also accompany patients to medical appointments, explain medical instructions to patients, and describe to the health-care provider limitations the patients may have in following a drug regimen, including the patient's side effects. In this study, Promotores are also part of the research group, acting as data collectors and providers of qualitative information for the researchers. In the TCM intervention, Promotores were autonomous agents, although closely affiliated to the HMA where the study was being conducted. A case manager who was part of the research team supervised the Promotores on a monthly basis, and the Promotores' salary was paid from research funds. This arrangement was convenient for the agencies, as the Promotore was not an employee of the HMA, the impact on the agency's budget was null, and the only expenses incurred by the agency was the time the Promotore spent with the case manager. This arrangement was expected to result in a net gain for the agency, as Promotores shared patient workload with case managers, due to the expected increase in patients' satisfaction related to perceived increase in care, and the potential decrease in disease episodes.

As part of the formative research needed to adapt the TCM project to the context of the HMA and their Hispanic patients, a preliminary assessment of the capacity of the HMAs to implement the project was conducted. The main findings were not unexpected. Most organizations lacked staff members linguistically and culturally attuned to the Hispanic HIV population, and had few educational materials appropriate to the literacy level of most Hispanic patients. The technical quality of the HIV medical care delivery in the HMAs was considered excellent, but the lack of culturally sensitive personnel and services hindered the access to quality care by Hispanics with limited English proficiency.

To test how well the TCM model assisted patients in managing their HIV disease and in avoiding costly medical emergencies, the research study was designed to answer five specific questions: (1) did the TCM model result in better quality of care for the patients; (2) did it result in increased patient satisfaction with their treatment; (3) did the model achieved better patient adherence to a treatment plan; (4) was the outcome of the model a decrease in emergency room visits and hospitalization days; and (5) were overall treatment costs smaller under the TCM model?

IMPLEMENTATION OF THE TCM MODEL

For the present study, the TCM-based intervention was implemented among a population of ambulatory adult HIV-seropositive Hispanic males, enrolled as patients in three New Mexico HMAs. Women were excluded from the study because the number of Hispanic women who were HIV-seropositive in the state was too small for any comparative analyses. The intervention was focused on this specific population because it has been demonstrated that when language and culture of patients differ from service providers, such factors serve as large barriers to HIV detection, treatment, and adherence to HAART regimens (Markson et al., 1998). Many health-care providers have some Spanish language ability, but are naïve about how patients' health-related cultural beliefs could influence treatment outcomes (Leininger, 1997; Murphy et al., 2003). Such is also true of many case managers who are serving patients who are recent immigrants, who are not yet proficient in English, and who are unfamiliar with medical terminology, even when addressed in Spanish. Given the large workloads of most HIV case managers, after the initial intake procedure the patient is typically seen monthly for a short amount of time, and mainly to schedule social services and medical appointments. These periodic encounters are brief, as the HIV case manager does not have the time to engage the patient in a long conversation. The Hispanic patient, being acculturated to a more passive role in a medical encounter and having language limitations, does not discuss medications' side effects, and the difficulties encountered in following instructions or the prescribed medical regimen. To help overcome these cultural and linguistic barriers to treatment, the chosen TCM Promotores were bilingual and bicultural. These two factors facilitate the job of Promotores when dealing with patients' problems, and when enlisting members of the patient's support network to help perform health-monitoring activities and foster the patients' adherence to medications.

STUDY METHODOLOGY AND DATA COLLECTION

The research study was set within one rural and two urban HIV Health Management Alliances (HMAs) in Northern and Southern New Mexico and within a non-profit organization (NGO), based in Ciudad Juarez, Mexico, that worked with the Southern HMA to provide continuity of social services for transborder HIV clients. In the latter case, these were clients who received medical services at the HMA and occasionally attended HIV support groups in Ciudad Juarez. The rural HMA was located in a town of about 45,293 people in the Northeast section of New Mexico, and served a county with a population of around 58,000 inhabitants. The urban HMAs served towns each with a population of around 120,000 inhabitants.

After an initial screening to establish their ethnic background, 125 patients were randomly assigned to an experimental or control group. Patients in the control group received the regular case management services, while patients in the experimental group, in addition to the regular case management care, received services from a TCM Promotore. Patients assigned to the intervention group received a more detailed explanation about the project, especially the role of Promotores as part of the HMA care team, and also about the need for periodic interviews with patients during the following two years. Participants assigned to the control group were told that a similar survey would be repeated in approximately 18 months.

Patients in both groups completed a 73-item 120-minute survey that had been developed and was proven to be reliable (alpha = .78) during the Promovisión pilot project. The survey included demographic and acculturation questions, and questions measuring adherence to HIV treatment; the number of opportunistic disease episodes, emergency room visits, hospitalization days in the previous year; and the level of satisfaction with their current HIV treatment. During the remainder of the project, constant observations and periodic interviews with Promotores, case managers, and patients in the experimental group were conducted to evaluate how well the intervention was being delivered. Towards the end of the project, patients in both groups completed a similar survey. Final summary interviews were conducted with all four Promotores, five case managers, and five available patients of the 24 remaining in the experimental group, to better understand the survey results, and to learn how to better implement similar projects in the future.

For the comparative qualitative data analysis of the interviews and observations, the NUD•IST qualitative analysis program was utilized to help organize thematically the perceptions of the participants about the quality of their treatment, continuity of health care, and disease episodes before and after implementation of the TCM. Although the use of a *t*-test was envisioned for the initial quantitative analysis of the pre- and post-surveys, unexpected problems with the data collection developed, and a *Wilcoxon's matched pairs* test was used instead. These problems are discussed in the following section.

THE REALITY OF FIELD RESEARCH

There were substantial changes in the initial data collection and analysis plan. After the project was underway, it was discovered that the random assignment of patients to the experimental and control groups had been corrupted. Against specific instructions by the researchers, case managers steered participants who were more compliant with the rules and regulations of the HMA to the control group to make the follow-up of that group easier to accomplish. This error transformed the study into a non-randomized design, and the control group was relabeled a comparison group. The initial patient assignment resulted in 60 patients being assigned to the intervention group and 65 to the comparison group.

Given the experience of the researchers in the Promovisión project, the attrition rate was expected to be small, but this proved to be a mistaken assumption. By the end of the project, the number of participants had decreased in the experimental group from the initial 60 to 24, and in the comparison group from 65 to 15. Structural changes unrelated to the research design and beyond the project team's control were the main causes of the high rate of attrition. Specifically, there were frequent changes at the executive level at two of the three HMAs, and the new directors had other priorities and were not as supportive of the project.

Another factor, paradoxically, was a result of the TCM project success. An increased sense of empowerment brought about by the Promotores' work and the project's participatory orientation caused some of the patients to feel that they did not need the Promotores' help any longer. At the beginning of the project, most patients could not conceive of returning to school or work, or becoming more socially engaged. As the project developed, many participants became more sociable, returned to work or school, and expanded their social support networks to include members of the newly-created Hispanic support groups. Follow-up phone interviews with some of the participants who dropped out of the intervention revealed that the work of the Promotores empowered them to get involved in other pursuits, and that the TCM project had become unnecessary and irrelevant to their new lifestyles.

FINDINGS

From the project onset, patients trusted Promotores to be their "peer advocates" who could represent their views to the HMA staff, and also bring them reliable information. This sense of trust was demonstrated by the amount of confidential information disclosed by patients about sexual practices, mental states, relationships, and the level of adherence to medications, and related to researchers during periodic interviews with Promotores.

During the active phase of the project, the Promotores established a routine that required contact with the patients assigned to them at least once a week during the first month and at regular intervals afterwards. Whenever needed, they visited participants at their homes, and if issues of confidentiality were at stake, they arranged for visits at a mutually acceptable place. Whenever a Promotore detected a possible health problem, or the participant requested a specific service, he consulted the case manager for the appropriate referral, and followed-up with the provider to ensure that the patient had complied with the referral or determine why not.

During the follow-up phase, access to patients became more difficult to the TCM research staff because of management and case managers' resistance to comply with the project research requirements. Access to medical chart data was very hard to obtain, which slowed down the final data collection and contributed to the low completion rate. This situation occurred before the inception of the HIPPA confidentiality process, which has made the data collection process even harder, albeit more secure.

Numerous barriers hindered data collection, and resulted in a limited number of patients participating in the final data collection, as well as in decreasing the power to conduct adequate analyses to detect statistically significant change for each of the five research questions. The results obtained, although not significant, were in the desired direction. The reported findings in the next section refer only to changes among patients in the experimental group, as conducting a comparative analysis would not have provided meaningful information.

The first research question examined whether the TCM would result in better quality of care to patients. Participants in the experimental group credited the Promotores with improving their relationships with their case managers, and reported that they were receiving better services, especially noting that their case managers were being informed of their needs and problems in a more timely fashion. Conversely, case managers were also positive about changes brought about by Promotores, especially by making them aware of the patients' perceptions of the case manager's role, and their help in overcoming language and cultural barriers, thus helping to improve the overall quality of services. Patients' personal experience with the Promotores was described as overwhelmingly positive. Patients felt safe to share personal stories knowing that likely the Promotore had had similar experiences, and could help them solve many problems, especially those dealing with medication side effects.

The second research question dealt with the degree of change in the participant's satisfaction with the services received from the HMA. The TCM Promotores' progress notes showed that participants reported more satisfaction with the services as their confidence increased in the quality of the HMA services. Patients perceived Promotores as being privileged to early information about new treatments and policies and, as a result, that they were receiving timely information. Patients also mentioned that they needed fewer services because they had become more autonomous and felt empowered to make decisions about their care. This finding is demonstrated by the results of the Wilcoxon's matched pairs test with 27 patients from the experimental group who were surveyed before and after the Promotores service. These patients had significantly decreased the number of times they visited the case manager ($z = -257$; $p = .010$), and had decreased the number of times they were asking for counseling ($z = -1.994$; $p = .046$). They were also in less need of stress management ($z = -2.081$; $p = 037$), visit to psychologists ($z = -2.023$; $p = .043$), or health-care help from friends ($z = -2.449$; $p = .014$). The number of responses from patients in the control group was too small to allow for any analysis.

Many times existing social support is removed when patients reveal their positive serostatus to family and friends. The stigma of being infected with HIV oftentimes isolates patients, and leaves them without the material and affective support that is essential for maintaining their quality of life. One of the strategies developed by Promotores to counteract this loss was the creation of support groups and informal social events to help increase the social support network of Hispanic patients. In the support groups Promotores provided knowledge about HIV services, side effects of specific medical regimens, and how to obtain access to health care, while the patients shared their own experiences and examples of strategies that worked and those that failed. Besides dealing with HIV treatment issues, discussions also involved issues dealing with family support, love, relationships, self-esteem, and planning for the future. The increased level of instrumental and emotional support necessary for participants' well-being, was especially important to recent immigrants who were far away from their support networks in their country of origin.

The third research question posited that patients enrolled in the TCM would report better adherence to the prescribed medication regimen. Patients reported a slight increase in the adherence to the medication regimen. Although there was no mechanism to validate the patients' reports, they stated that strategies to comply with the medication regimen helped them become more disciplined about their medical care, and especially more aware of their medication schedules. In addition, the increased social contact with other participants promoted more discussions about how to deal with personal and institutional barriers to adherence to the demanding HAART medication regimen. Patients reported sharing strategies to mask their serostatus to others who might see them taking medications at regular intervals. They became more cognizant of medications' side effects and planned to take their medications at times when they would not interfere with their activities.

The results of the fourth research question concerned changes in morbidity and looked for evidence that the TCM project resulted in fewer visits to emergency rooms and fewer hospitalization days. At the end of the project, the number of hospitalizations reported by patients in the experimental group had decreased by 7% over a period of 18 months. Moreover, participants also reported that visits to hospital emergency rooms during the same period decreased from 1.84 to 0.74 or a 40% decrease per participant. Given the small number of patients contacted for the follow-up test, and the lack of a validation mechanism for these claims, neither of these results could be described to have resulted in verifiable cost-savings.

The final research question examined if better adherence to treatment, fewer hospitalization days, better continuity of care, and more participant satisfaction justified the added cost of the TCM model. Not enough data was available to reliably answer this question. The project had to rely on the participant's best recollection of medical costs, because access to participant charts and financial data was impeded at the end of the project. From data provided by patients, the average number of hospitalization days in the beginning of the project was 17.5 days per year. In the last year of the project, hospitalization days decreased to 10 per year, resulting in a cumulative decrease of about 200 hospitalization days. Given that hospitalization of an HIV patient in New Mexico averages about $2,000 a day, this may have resulted in cost savings of about $200,000 over the course of the study. Unfortunately, such a claim cannot be substantiated, given the lack of verifiable hospitalization expenses.

DISCUSSION: LESSONS LEARNED

Most of the barriers that impeded the completion of the envisioned data collection and analysis to evaluate how well the TCM intervention had fared, were due to institutional and research project issues: significant personnel changes in the HMAs, and the time it took researchers to become aware of the impact of these changes in accomplishing the tasks requested by the research protocol.

Unpredictable changes in the HMA management and staff, and the necessity of obtaining continued cooperation of each newly-hired case manager and executive staff to continue the project was not always successful. One of the HMAs dropped out of the project completely, and the management of the other two HMAs became less cooperative and made access to the patients' medical information hard to obtain. The willingness of HMA agencies to devote resources to the project decreased after the initial period. This event was a direct result of the unforeseen increase in case manager workload because the planned shift of some of the case managers' workload to Promotores did not occur. This situation was unforeseen, the direct result of the increased amount of care delivered to the patients by the Promotores who were bringing new problems to the attention of case managers. Most of these newly articulated problems were related to access to agency resources, and for some time they were solved by the formation of Hispanic support groups. Albeit desirable, one unforeseen development beyond the researchers' control was the Hispanic patients' increased sense of empowerment and the demands placed on the HMAs for services that they perceived were being denied them. Increased requests for services created tensions with case managers who became less interested in cooperating with the Promotores in facilitating access to patients and to data.

The decline of interest in the project by case managers and the HMA management was understandable as the short-term payoff for the agencies did not materialize. Given the HMA's changing short-term priorities due to budgetary changes and other management issues, the Promotores' request for data and increased access to case managers was deemed too onerous by the same case managers who were supportive of the project at the beginning. This situation translated into an increased unwillingness by new case managers to fully support the Promotores' effort. The great distances between research sites, coupled with the researchers not being constantly present to immediately resolve problems, and dissatisfaction with the project were not addressed in a timely manner and worsened to the point that remedial steps to correct them were hard to implement.

The geographical distribution of the three sites in the state required that researchers relied heavily on the Promotores for data collection. Promotores complained about the constant demand for data by the researchers, and felt that the time used for data collection was being "taken away" from the time they should dedicate to the patients. At the beginning of the project the Promotores received training to better sensitize them to the nature of research projects and the need of reliable data analysis, but given the distances between all three sites, there was not consistent monitoring of data collection, except for visits to the three sites by the project manager on a monthly basis. The main lesson learned from this experience involves the need to have a budgeted, permanent project manager on-site who is responsible for the day-to-day activities of the project, especially when the sites are so distant; or it may be necessary to restrict the research to sites that can be visited in a single day trip. Data from the site within 50 miles of the researchers' main location was collected with fewer problems, except for those caused by changes in the agency's case managers and executive management.

Another large barrier that impeded the timely collection of data was related to issues with the clients' privacy. Although they were willing to participate in the project, most rural and some urban clients did not want to have the Promotore visit them at their homes to complete the surveys. This situation made the completion of the final questionnaires very difficult to schedule.

Finally, the data collection problem at the end of the intervention can be attributed to the success of the Promotores' efforts to foster a sense of self-reliance among patients. Because one of the TCM project objectives was to encourage participants to become more independent and active, their daily schedules became busier with more social meetings, work and school obligations. The speed with which these lifestyle changes occurred was not foreseen by researchers, as this component in the Promovisión project was not as successful. The lesson for future research is that faster development in the expected changes among participants may bring about other changes that may interfere with data collection. Researchers have to be prepared for the fallout from increased success as well as failures. Constant monitoring of unexpected developments and timely reaction to them is crucial for the success of a research project.

IMPROVEMENTS

One of the most important results of the intervention was the increased self-reliance demonstrated by the patients. For most patients, the Promotores became role models and an exemplar of the possibility that many HIV patients could return to work and make substantial contributions to the community. In addition, Promotores were perceived as individuals who by virtue of their engagement with other patients and patients' families had a more satisfying social life. This observation made the clients start to question their "sick" role, to become involved in more social activities, and to start to entertain the possibility that they themselves could have part-time jobs and consider returning to school for further training.

The creation and maintenance of the Hispanic support groups were another successful accomplishment of the TCM intervention. The realization that there were other HIV-positive Hispanics interested in openly discussing their experiences in living with HIV, provided patients with a safe place to express their problems and to look jointly for solutions. In these groups, patients became more socially active and started networking with other patients who were already working. This situation resulted in the rise in the number of patients who became employed and who were once more taking control of their lives. Once more, the success in this component had unforeseen results. The patients' increased social life and ability to reenter the job world, over time, decreased their attendance at the HIV support groups. Follow-up with patients, who were initially active in the support groups and social gatherings, revealed that they had formed smaller social groups with fellow patients based on shared interests, and had continued to socialize on a regular basis. They described these gatherings as a "meeting of friends," and not as a support group.

While the barriers for accomplishing the planned research goals were substantial and the statistical results of the research questions were not significant, there were marked improvements brought about by the TCM intervention, and with further development it could become a successful model for improving the level of care of Hispanic HIV-positive patients.

The program also demonstrated that Promotores not only brought together clients and case managers, but also helped the patients' friends, family, and partners become more involved in the HIV care process. In the United States, in most instances, family members are not invited to become involved in the HIV patient care unless a crisis develops and they are needed to make decisions for a patient. Hispanic families, on the other hand, expect to be more directly involved with the medical care of their members. Although the stigma of the disease may separate family members from the HIV patient, those who decide to help will become involved in increasing the quality of life of the patients. Promotores acted as counselors for family members, explaining the disease, dispelling myths about contagion and helping to quell the fear of the disease. Promotores also informally trained caregivers to help monitor the health status of patients, to detect negative changes brought about by medications, and taught them how to access medical care before an avoidable crisis developed.

IMPLICATIONS FOR FUTURE RESEARCH

Further research to test the model in community-based organizations dealing with HIV/AIDS should concentrate in testing the cost effectiveness of the model and the feasibility of the program sustainability. It is recommended that a similar research protocol be implemented either in HIV care agencies that are nearer each other, or by local research teams that could maintain a closer supervision of the data collection mechanisms. The randomization could be made at the agency level to avoid the problems encountered during the initial patient assignment. Instead of obtaining memoranda of understanding, a more formal and specific memoranda of commitment between the research organization and the HIV care agencies should be drafted listing in precise terms the expectations of both agencies, the commitment of both groups to the success of the research, and the continuing support to the endeavor by future managers. The provision of a monetary incentive to the agencies at the beginning of the project to offset any expenses that may be caused by the research would further solidify their commitment to the project.

Although the management teams of the HMAS were not as supportive during the last phase of the research, they recognized that the program had a positive impact in their agencies. The training of HIV-positive individuals as Promotores provided them with a set of valuable communication skills and strategies to employ those skills to help improve the quality of life of other patients. The value of Promotores to the agencies became evident when, after the research funding ended, all three Promotores were hired at their original agencies to perform the same functions they had during the TCM model intervention.

REFERENCES

Bozzette, S. A., Joyce G., McCaffrey, D. F., Leibowitz, A. A., Morton, S. C., Berry S. H. et al. (2001). Expenditures for the care of HIV-infected patients in the era of Highly Active Antiretroviral Therapy. *JAMA*, *344* (11): 817-823.

Chabot, E. A. (1987). Primary health care is not cheap: A case study from Guinea Bissau. *International Journal of Health Services*, *17*: 1411-1417.

Chesney, M. A. (2000). Factors affecting adherence to antiretroviral therapy. *Clinical Infectious Diseases*, *30*: S171-S17.

Fleishman, J. A. (1997). Utilization of home care among people with HIV infection. *Health Services Research, 32* (2): 155-75.

Freire, P. L. (1970). *Pedagogy of the oppressed.* New York: Herder and Herder.

Friedland, J., Renwick, R., & Mccoll, M. (1996). Coping and social support as determinants of quality of life in HIV/AIDS. *AIDS Care 8* (1): 15-3.

Giblin, P. T. (1989). Effective utilization and evaluation of indigenous health care workers. *Public Health Reports, 104*: 361-368.

Health Maintenance Alliance: New Mexico's HIV/AIDS Health Management Alliances (2004). Mexico AIDS Education and Training Center, University of New Mexico Health Sciences Center. Retrieved on September 10, 2004 from http://www.aidsinfonet.org/articles.php?articleID = 810

Hellinger, F. J. (1998) Cost and financing of care for persons with HIV disease: An overview. *Health Care Financing Review, 19*(3): 1-14.

Krantz, R. S. (2003). The patient-provider relationship and adherence to highly active antiretroviral therapy (HAART). International Association of Physicians in AIDS Care. *Elements of success: An international conference on adherence to antiretroviral therapy,* December 4-7, 2003, Dallas, Texas, USA. Retrieved on June 20, 2005 from http://www.iapac.org/

Leininger, M. (1997). Transcultural nursing: Scientific and humanistic care discipline. *Journal of Trans-cultural Nursing, 8* (2), 54-55.

Leserman, J., Petitto, J. M., Golden, R. N., Gaynes, B. N., Gu, H., Perkins D. O. et al. (2000). Impact of stressful life events, depression, social support, coping, and cortisol on progression to AIDS. *American Journal of Psychiatry, 157*: 1221-1228.

Markson, L. E., Houchens, R., Fanning, T. R., & Turner, B. J. (1998). Repeated emergency department use by HIV-infected persons: Effect of clinic accessibility and expertise in HIV care. *Journal of Acquired Immune Deficiency Syndromes & Human Retrovirology, 17* (1): 35-41.

McDonnell, M., DiIorio, C., McCarty, F., Yeager, K., Wang, T., Iverson, H. et al. (2003). Antiretroviral medication complexity and adherence. International Association of Physicians in AIDS Care. *Elements of success: An international conference on adherence to antiretroviral therapy,* December 4-7, 2003, Dallas, Texas, USA. Retrieved on June 2005 from http://www.iapac.org/

Murphy, D. A., Roberts, J. K., Hoffman, D., Molina, A., & Lu, M. C. (2003). Barriers and successful strategies to antiretroviral adherence among HIV-infected monolingual Spanish-speaking patients. *AIDS Care, 15* (2): 217-230.

Murphy, E. L., Collier, A. C., Kalish, L. A., Assmann, S. F., Para, M. F., Flanigan, T. P. et al. (2001). Highly Active Antiretroviral Therapy decreases mortality and morbidity in patients with advanced HIV disease. *Annals of Internal Medicine, 135* (1): 17-26.

Palella, F. J. Jr., Delaney, K. M., Moorman, A. C., Loveless, M. O., Fuhrer, J., Satten, G. A. et al. (1998). Declining morbidity and mortality among patients with advanced human immunodeficiency virus infection. HIV outpatient study. *New England Journal of Medicine, 338* (13): 853-60.

Ramos, R. L., & Ferreira-Pinto, J. B. (2002). Successful capacity building for community based organizations. *AIDS Education and Prevention, 14* (3): 196-205.

Ramos, R. L., Hernandez, A., Ferreira-Pinto, J. B., Ortiz, M., & Gallegos, G. (2006) Promovisión: Designing a capacity-building program to strengthen and expand the role of Promotores in HIV prevention. *Health Promotion Practice, 7*: 444-449.

Schackman, B. R., Freedberg, K. A., Weinstein, M. C., Sax, P. E., Losina, E., Zhang, H. et al. (2002). Cost-effectiveness implications of the timing of antiretroviral therapy in HIV-infected adults. *Archives of Internal Medicine, 162*: 2478-2486.

Scholl, E. (1985). An assessment of community health workers in Nicaragua. *Social Science and Medicine, 20*: 207-214.

Stasiak, D. (1991). Culture care theory with Mexican-Americans in an urban context. In M. Leininger (Ed.), *Culture care diversity and universality: A theory of nursing* (pp. 79-203). New York: National League of Nursing Press.

Wang, I. L. (1975). Training of the barefoot doctor in the People's Republic of China from prevention to curative services. *International Journal of Health Services, 5*: 475-488.

Warrick, L. H., Wood, A. H., Meister, J. S., & de Zapien, J. G. (1992). Evaluation of peer health worker prenatal outreach program for Hispanic farm worker families. *Journal of Community Health, 17*: 13-26.

doi:10.1300/J187v05n02_10

Glossary

Acculturation	Sociocultural changes that take place when individuals originating in one culture move to a different one. Such changes imply the degree to which an individual assimilates, identifies with, and takes on the lifestyle, culture and language of the new country of residence. These reported studies refer to the degree to which Mexican origin persons change when faced with the situation of living in a cultural context differing from their own (Padilla & Perez, 2003).
AIDS	A person with HIV and a T-cell count of less than 200 is considered to have a diagnosis of AIDS, Acquired Immune Deficiency Syndrome (Arizona AETC, 2003).
Bilingual	Persons who speak two languages; in these studies the languages are English and Spanish.
Bi-sexual	An individual who is both heterosexual and homosexual; who has active and passive sexual interests in both genders (Dorland, 1995).
CdV	Abbreviation for title of New Mexico AIDS service agency, Camino de Vida, English translation is: "Path or Road to Life."

[Haworth co-indexing entry note]: "Glossary." Co-published simultaneously in *Journal of HIV/AIDS & Social Services* (The Haworth Press, Inc.) Vol. 5, No. 2, 2006, pp. 159-164; and: *Outreach and Care Approaches to HIV/AIDS Along the US-Mexico Border* (ed: Herman Curiel, and Helen Land) The Haworth Press, Inc., 2006, pp. 159-164. Single or multiple copies of this article are available for a fee from The Haworth Document Delivery Service [1-800-HAWORTH, 9:00 a.m. - 5:00 p.m. (EST). E-mail address: docdelivery@haworthpress.com].

Available online at http://jhaso.haworthpress.com
© 2006 by The Haworth Press, Inc. All rights reserved.
doi:10.1300/J187v05n02_11

Centro Nacional para la Prevencion y el control del VIH/SIDA	English translation: National Center for the Prevention & Control of HIV/AIDS; serves as the national center for Mexico.
Colonia	Informal Spanish-language word for neighborhood or settlement.
Elisa testing	Considered the gold standard for preliminary HIV testing. Detects serum antibodies to HIV (Nassar, Keiser, & Gregg, 2004).
Epidemiology	Study of disease patterns and distribution in human groups (De la Torre & Estrada, 2001).
Focus group	A group formed to help develop the research questions, or as a form of non-probability sampling (Marlow & Boone, 2005).
Gay male	Label used for males whose primary sexual orientation is homosexual who show active or passive interests in persons of the same sex.
HIV seropositive	Refers to individuals who test positive for having the Human Immune virus that survives by attaching itself to receptive immune system T-cells also referred to as CD-4 cells. As cells are destroyed individual becomes vulnerable to infections (Arizona AETC).
Homeopathic meds	Use of pharmacist to prescribe medications. A common practice among US/Mexico populations with limited access to formal health.
Homosexual	A person who is sexually attracted to persons of the same sex (Dorland, 1995).
HOW	Title abbreviation given to health outreach workers, selected because of their peer status and similar gender or sexual orientation to target population.
IDU	Abbreviation used by staff with HIV/AIDS organizations to refer to person's route of virus transmission, intravenous drug use.
Jornalero	A Spanish word for day laborer.

Latino/Hispanic	Terms used interchangeably to refer to persons with ethnic heritage by birth or ancestors from a Spanish-speaking country.
Lesbian	Label for a female homosexual who shows active or passive sexual interest in other females.
Matrix	One method of developing a classification system in the analysis of qualitative data.
Maquiladora	Term used to refer to mechanized assembly plants located along the US/Mexico border that employ Mexican workers for low wages.
Mexican	A person whose nationality or citizenship is Mexican.
Mexican origin	A person who was born in Mexico or who has one or both parents or ancestors who came from Mexico.
Migrant	A person who migrates, in context of reported study, from Mexico to the United States for work. These migrants may be legal or undocumented. It is implied that the period of residence in any one place is contingent on finding work.
MSM	MSM refers collectively to men who have sex with men for purpose of identifying HIV routes of virus exposure. This category does not distinguish heterosexuals from gay or bi-sexual males.
Ora-Sure test	Rapid HIV test with use of saliva. Western Blot referred to as "gold standard" test is used to verify diagnosis (Arizona AETC, 2003).
Peer advocates	In context of HIV/AIDS care, peer advocates are usually part-time staff affected by HIV who use their personal disease knowledge to educate peers in prevention. Normally these individuals are assigned roles in outreach to at-risk peers; some conduct Ora-sure HIV tests in the field and help educate newly diagnosed individuals about HIV and care protocols.

Primary prevention

Educational activities designed to reach at-risk populations to prevent exposure to HIV.

Projecto

Spanish word for project.

Promotor/Promotora

English translation for concept role is promoter. In Latin American countries, a promotora (feminine noun) is an indigenous unpaid volunteer person who receives training through a formal health-care institution to help promote health prevention activities and provide a community link for professional care providers.

Qualitative research

Qualitative researchers use observation to examine particulars of a phenomenon to describe relationships among particulars. Qualitative information involves the non-numerical examination of phenomena, using words instead of numbers (Marlow & Boone, 2005).

Quantitative research

The goal of the quantitative approach to science is to search for causes of phenomena. The quantitative approach requires studying large numbers of subjects, because the central concern is ability to generalize the results (Marlow & Boone, 2005).

Random assignment

The research process by which every subject has an equal chance of being assigned to a control group or a treatment group.

Ryan White Care Act

Enacted in 1990, the Ryan White Comprehensive AIDS Resources Emergency (CARE) Act provides federal funds to support primary medical care and support services for persons living with HIV/AIDS.

Secondary prevention

Efforts to treat patients early to prevent progression of the disease (Timmreck, 1997).

Sex worker

A person of either gender who has sex for money.

Social stigma	Social stigma is a function of having an attribute such as HIV/AIDS that conveys a devalued social identity in a particular context (Crocker, Major, & Steele, 1998).
Tertiary prevention	Treatment to slow or stop progression of HIV to minimize care required (Timmreck, 1997).
Trans-border populations	Persons who have access to cross the U.S.-Mexico border regularly.
U.S.-Mexico border region	An area demarcated by the geo-political boundary between the United States and Mexico. As defined in 1983 by the La Paz Agreement between the United States and Mexico, this region extends 62 miles (100 km) north and south of the border and extends 1,863 miles (~3,000 km) from California to Texas.
Vicios	A Spanish word that refers to acquired habits.
Western blot	Confirmatory HIV test that detects antibodies to individual HIV proteins and glycoproteins that have been separated into discrete bands by electrophoresis (Nassar, Keiser, & Gregg, 2004).

REFERENCES

Arizona AIDS Education & Training Center (2003). *HIV & AIDS: A self-paced training manual.* Tucson, AZ: University of Arizona Health Sciences Center.

Crocker, J., Major, B., & Steele, C. (1998). Social stigma. In. D. T. Gilbert, S. T. Fiske, & G. Lindzey (Eds.), *The handbook of social psychology* (pp. 504-553). New York: McGraw-Hill.

De la Torre, A., & Estrada, A. (2001). *Mexican Americans & health.* Tucson, AZ: University of Arizona Press.

Dorland, N. W. (1995). *Dorland's pocket medical dictionary* (25th ed.). Philadelphia, PA: W. B. Saunders Co.

Marlow, C. R., & Boone, S. (2005). *Research methods for generalist social work.* Belmont, CA: Brooks/Cole-Thomson Learning.

Nassar, N. N., Keiser, P., & Gregg, C. R. (2004). *Parkland pocket guide to HIV care* (3rd ed.). Dallas, TX: Texas/Oklahoma AIDS Education & Training Center, 22-23.

Padilla, A. M., & Perez, W. (2003). Acculturation, social identity, and social cognition: A new perspective. *Hispanic Journal of Behavioral Sciences, 25,* 35-55.

WEBSITE RESOURCES

AETC National Resource Center:
http://www.aidsetc.org/

Border Epidemiology and Environmental Health Center:
http://www.nmsu.edu/ %7Ebec/index.html

Centers for Disease Control and Prevention:
http://www.cdc.gov/

HRSA HIV/AIDS Bureau:
http://www.hab.hrsa.gov/

JOHNS HOPKINS AIDS Services:
http://www.hopkins-aids.edu/

The Measurement Group (HIV/AIDS Program Evaluations):
http://www.themeasurementgroup.com/

US-Mexico Border Health Association:
http://www.usmbha.org/

Index

© 2006 by The Haworth Press, Inc. All rights reserved.

Printed and bound by CPI Group (UK) Ltd, Croydon, CR0 4YY

17/10/2024

01775687-0020